THE
JAMAICAN
HANDBOOK
FOR THE
ELDERLY

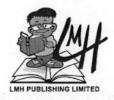

LMH PUBLISHING LIMITED

A number of agencies have helped in the production, such as the Ministry of Social Security and the National Council for Senior Citizens. In compiling the book the publishers have used fairly widely Wesley J. Smith, The Senior Citizens' Handbook, published by Price Stern Stone and have contacted them for permission.

Special thanks to Ms. K. Denise Henry, Legal Estate Planner, for the section "Putting your affairs in order".

Cover Design: Sanya Dockery
Design & Typesetting: Michelle M. A. Mitchell

Published by: LMH Publishing Ltd.
Suite 10-11
Sagicor Industrial Park
7 Norman Road
Kingston C.S.O; Jamaica
Tel: 876-938-0005
Fax: 876-928-8036
Email: lmhbookpublishing@cwjamaica.com
Website: www.lmhpublishing.com

Printed in the USA   ISBN: 978-976-8202-73-4

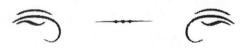

Dedication

To all the elderly people in
Jamaica and the Caribbean.

"Elder" - *An older person; one's senior.*

       - *A senior member of a tribe,*
        who has influence or authority.

Source: Collins Dictionary of the
English Language,
Second Edition

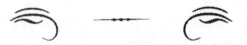

CONTENTS

- General safety tips
- Maintaining a proper posture

- Personal hygiene
- Garbage disposal
- Regular spring cleaning

- Lifestyle extension tips
- Types of work environments that optimize health
- Spiritual health

2 What You Should Know About Your Medical Care

3 To Stay Or To GO

4 Dealing With The Not So Pleasant Aspects Of The Golden Years

5 Money Matters and Employment

- Certificates of deposits - description, risks and earning potentials
- Government bonds
- Corporate bonds
- Stocks
- Mutual funds
- Trust deeds

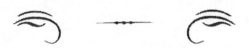

FOREWORD

The Jamaican Handbook for the Elderly is both a needed and timely publication. The over 60 years old or senior citizen population is the fastest growing segment of the population in the world and also here in Jamaica. The present population of over 250,000 persons is expected to double over the next thirty years, at a time when ageing is being seen in a new light. Old age is no longer automatically associated with illness and incapacity, but is now seen as a lifelong event over which individuals have some amount of control and have to assume responsibility for.

The importance of this book cannot be overstressed, as it not only embraces the concept of active ageing in a very practical way, but it also helps the reader to make informed decisions about several aspects of their lives, which can have an impact on the quality. The emphasis on social and financial planning and decision making, including the very important section on housing and accommodation is a fresh approach, especially as it relates to our local situation. It focuses our attention on other aspects of planning that will become necessary in later years.

The book in its final chapters includes suggestions on topics often thought of as unpleasant, but which are a reality of life that many senior citizens face. These include violence, abuse and death.

Finally, it is often said that *'prevention is better than cure'*. The book also has some useful advice as it relates to preventive medicine.

The National Council for Senior Citizens endorses its publication and recommends that it be read by everyone.

Dr. Denise Eldemire-Shearer
Chairman
National Council for Senior Citizens

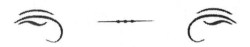

INTRODUCTION

Ageing is a part and parcel of everyone's experience. It is a process that we cannot control. What we can control, however, are the preparations and choices that we make as we approach the golden years.

It is often said, that *'with age comes wisdom'*. For those of us who are blessed with the former and not the latter, this book has a wealth of information that will effectively educate us on how to approach this rather exciting, but challenging stage of our lives.

It is divided into five chapters, which cover such areas as maintaining health, employment, money matters, accommodation and the not so pleasant aspects of the golden years, among others. It is hoped that as you read this book, you will not only be educated on the various choices and challenges that senior citizens face, but having done so, you will be more informed when making decisions that will affect the rest of your life.

Remember, 'age is just a number', but with it comes wisdom!

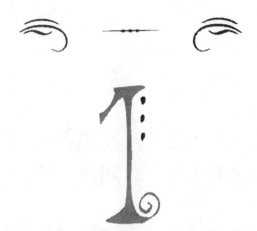

KEEPING YOUNG
AND HEALTHY

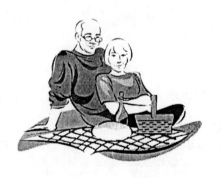

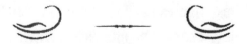

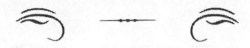

UNDERSTANDING THE AGEING PROCESS

Ageing is defined as a lifelong developmental process of physical, social and psychological changes.

Why should the human body give out after 70, 80, or even 120 years? Why are older people more susceptible to diseases, more inclined to have impaired vision and hearing, and more likely to lose some of the physical and mental capacity they once enjoyed?

There are no satisfactory answers to these questions. Although we are mortals, it is possible that in the future human beings could live much longer lives. The present potential life span for human beings is said to be 115 years and today thousands of people live to be over 100. Jamaicans now expect to live an average of 75 years. Women have a life expectancy of 78 years and men 73 years. Yet these figures have very little to do with potential life expectancy, as most people have their lives altered or shortened by diseases and disabilities, rather than the natural process of ageing.

A lot is known about diseases that affect people and cause death. Much less is known about the ageing process, as it involves quite complex cell processes. However, this mystery of life is being unravelled and will offer opportunities that were once considered to be only possible in science fiction.

Your life literally depends upon the ability of your cells to regenerate. They do this in a manner similar to one-cell organisms that simply divide and go on living as two "daughter" one-cell organisms. Before your cells can divide to reproduce themselves, they must first produce a duplicate copy of the genes. One of the most important examples of replication is that of the red blood cells. The red blood cells live only an average of 110 days, and they must be constantly replaced. Without replacement, you could develop anemia. The lining of the small intestine is completely replaced every three days. The skin is constantly regenerated with the new cells formed in the deeper layers, which is called the dermis, while the old cells move to the top, which is called the epidermis, and are shed. It is the constant regeneration of these cells that keeps the body young and helps it to heal itself after an injury.

Why the body does not continue to renew itself indefinitely so we do not grow old? There are a number of theories for this big question:

- The regeneration process is under the control of a

genetic script, which determines when certain events in your life should occur. For example, the onset of menopause.

- Organs and tissues often undergo changes because the cells used to form them no longer function in the same manner that they once did when they were young. For example, ovaries are not activated until puberty arrives. As we age, their functions begin to slow down and eventually cease completely.

- Some investigators believe that the immune system is responsible for ageing. As people get older, their bodies produce more autoimmune antibodies. Sometimes these antibodies attack the tissues of the body as if they were foreign substances or bacteria. In extreme states they may cause such autoimmune diseases as rheumatoid arthritis and thyroid disease. Additionally, the body's immune defences may decrease with age. The thymus gland, which prepares white blood cells and act as a defence mechanism to protect the body, gradually deteriorates. The decrease in rheumatoid can result in someone becoming more susceptible to diseases, such as pneumonia. In other words, the body just stops functioning.

There are other theories such as the "free-radical" theory and the "cross-linked" theory that describe what happens, but do not explain why. But perhaps a theory explaining why the body ages is not the most important key to unlocking the mystery of longevity. After all, it is not old age that kills or alters our lives, but the many diseases that affect us.

Senile Dementia

This refers to the severe loss of mental ability that some people experience as they age, which results in that person being totally incapacitated and no longer in touch with reality. Medical science now recognizes that senile dementia is not a condition that develops as a result of the ageing process; rather it is as a result of the many diseases that afflict us. Scientists are now trying to unravel the mystery of diseases, rather than the mystery of ageing as a means of preventing and treating senile dementia. However, it is possible that as researchers begin to figure out the complex interrelationship between nerve cells and brain chemistry, they may also discover the reasons as to why we age.

The ageing Brain

Often it is not ageing, but disuse of the brain that results in decreased mental functions, especially as we age. It is important to note that maintaining one's ability to concentrate, and continuous stimulation of memory with tasks and problem solving are essential for the mental aspect of the brain to function at its best. Whereas the brain may continue to regulate your blood pressure and heart rate and determines whether or not you sweat, if you do not use it for mental tasks, its ability to remember will decrease from lack of use rather than age.

Sexual Function

Estrogen keeps a woman's sexual organs in a state of readiness. Loss of this hormone, which occurs with age, will not cause her sexual interest to disappear but will certainly influence her interest in sex. This problem is easily remedied by oestrogen replacement therapy.

In the healthy older male, cessation of testosterone production is not an issue as the testicles continue to produce high levels of this hormone throughout life. Instead, the failure to perform sexually or to have an erection is usually a result of poor circulation due to disease, or to changes in the nerve fibres controlling erections, or to the side effects of some medication.

The Sense Organs

The special senses, such as hearing, seeing and tasting, are extensions of the nervous system. The progressive loss of taste, smell and hearing could be caused by the ageing of the end cells of the related organ, such as the taste buds in the mouth or the olfactory cells in the nose. But it could also be that they were damaged because of illness or some form of disease. The maintenance of these functions at optimal levels may depend on both preventing or curing disease and preventing ageing of the sense cells.

The Heart

Very little is known about ageing of the heart. Coronary heart disease that results in heart attacks is not caused by ageing at all but by diseases that involve the arteries of the heart muscle. Genetic factors play a role as they can influence a person's cholesterol level, thus increasing their risks of developing blocked arteries. In addition, many older people develop 'weak' hearts because that organ has not been exercised enough. This is largely due to the reduction in physical activity as they age.

The Muscles and Skeleton

The changes in the muscle and skeleton are another area where disease and disuse are often confused with age. There is some loss of muscle fibres caused by the degeneration of some of the nerve cells (due to age), which control them. However, exercise can maintain, strengthen and enlarge the remaining muscle tissue. As it relates to the bones, their structure is continuously changing. It should be noted though that after the age of 30 years, more bone mass is lost that is formed and this results in a gradual decrease in the size of the skeleton.

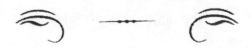

MAINTAINING HEALTH

Seneca (4BC - 65 AD) in giving his views on maintaining health, vitality and living longer lives, stated best when he emphasized the need to eat moderate amounts of well-balanced foods, get plenty of fresh air and exercise, and to live a stress-free lifestyle. These factors do influence our quality of life, as they provide the necessary defense against disease and ensure that our bodies are kept in good condition.

NUTRITION

<u>Eating Habits</u>

The life span of the average Jamaican has dramatically increased over the past century. Unfortunately, knowledge of our changing nutritional needs as we age has not kept pace. In addition, surveys have shown that people who are healthy and live longer have traditionally been light eaters. They never overeat. They quit before they are full, and they always leave the table feeling slightly hungry.

Currently, too many seniors are undernourished as a result of:

- Ageing
- Eating processed foods low in nutritional value
- Reduced metabolism
- Diminished appetite (due to depression or loneliness, among others)
- Effects of medication
- Lack of cooking skills (especially in widowers)
- Dental problems

In addition, most senior citizens do not realize that their nutritional needs change as they age. The following are some of the changes that occur as we age and their nutritional significance.

- Older people produce less saliva and often have poor dentures. This causes difficulty with very dry foods.
- An estimated 30% of seniors lose their ability to produce stomach acid. This interferes with the absorption of some nutrients, such as vitamin B 12 and folic acid. Deficiencies in these nutrients, as well as vitamin B6, can cause neurological changes,

such as decreased alertness, loss of memory and numbness in the extremities.

- The reduction of the natural movement of food and enzyme activity in the gastrointestinal tract, known to be associated with ageing, often results in difficulties in the digestion of certain foods. Also, this reduction in the natural movement of food through the intestines causes food to remain in the intestines for a longer period of time, thus producing harder stools and constipation.

- ageing affects certain senses, such as taste, smell and vision, which often affect the types of food that are chosen. Salt and sweet taste sensations can dramatically decrease with age, with the result that the elderly may opt for more richly seasoned foods. The problem is that some spicy foods produce gas. Consequently, many older persons will experience "heartburn" that is often caused by the production of gas rather than increased acidity. In order to compensate for the gradual loss of taste, others may resort to using extra salt, in which case may result in the retention of water and high blood pressure.

- As we age, we need less of some minerals (such as sodium which lowers blood pressure) and more of others (such as calcium for bone mass).

- Because of changes in the body and decreased physical activity, older people usually need the same amount of nutrients but fewer calories, as the rate at which the body uses energy tends to decrease. For some, food intake is generally lower, and the amount of lean body tissues decreases while the amount of body fat increases. Yet, others maintain old eating habits, not realizing that most people gain weight as they age.

Nutrients - What They Are

A nutrient is a substance that promotes bodily growth or improvement and repairs the damages caused by everyday 'wear and tear'. The following are the nutrients that are needed for the maintenance of good health and well-being.

1. *Carbohydrates* include starches, sugars and dietary fibre. Starches and sugar supply the body with energy. Dietary fibre provides bulk in the diet, which encourages regular bowel movement.

2. *Fats* provide energy and are carriers of fat-soluble vitamins. Some fats are used in the formation of cell membranes and hormones. This nutrient also adds flavour to foods.

3. *Proteins* are the building blocks of the body. They are needed for growth and maintenance as well as for the replacement of body cells. Proteins are an essential ingredient of enzymes and hormones

whose function it is to regulate body processes. Any extra protein is metabolized to produce energy or is converted into body fat and stored as energy.

4. *Vitamins* are organic substances needed by the body in trace quantities. They do not supply energy, but assist in the release of energy from energy-rich compounds such as carbohydrates, fats and protein. Vitamins also stimulate chemical reactions in the body.

5. *Minerals* are also needed in relatively small amounts and do not supply energy. They build strong bones and teeth and are a component of haemoglobin found in red blood cells. Minerals help maintain body fluids and are necessary ingredients for certain chemical reactions in the body.

6. *Water* is often called the "forgotten nutrient." It is needed to replace the water lost from the body during sweating and urination. In addition, water helps to transport nutrients throughout the body, removes waste and regulates the body's temperature.

Major Food Groups And Their Nutrients

Adults over 50 years old need more of some nutrients and less of others. Vitamins and minerals optimize their healing potential and it is important that their diet consist of:

- *Fruits and Vegetables*

  These provide vitamins, minerals and dietary fibre. They also provide starch and protein. Fruits with skin and edible seeds are especially rich in fibre and deep-yellow vegetables are good sources of vitamins A. Dark-green vegetables are a good source of vitamins A and C, riboflavin, folic acid, iron, calcium, magnesium and potassium. Fruits, such as melons, oranges, grapefruits, tangerines and lemons are rich in vitamin C and calcium. These two nutrients can also be found in greens such as garden cherries, guavas, kale and callaloo. Almost all vegetables and fruits are low in fat, and none contain cholesterol.

- *Breads, Cereals, Rice and Pastas*

  Foods in this group provide starch, thiamine, riboflavin, niacin, iron, magnesium, folacin, fibre and protein.

- *Meat, Poultry, Fish and Beans*

  It is important that you vary your food selection and this group offers a distinct nutritional advantage. Red meat, for instance, is a good source of zinc. Liver and egg yolks, although high in cholesterol, are valuable sources of vitamins. Dry beans, peas, soybeans and nuts are good sources of magnesium. All foods of animal origin contain vitamin B12, while foods of vegetable origin do not.

- *Fats, Oils, Sweets and Alcohol*

   Most foods in this group provide relatively low levels of vitamins, minerals and protein, but are high in calories. Vegetable oils, however, do supply a good amount of vitamin E and essential fatty acids.

Tips For Good Nutrition

As one gets older, the chances of becoming ill are greater, and health experts believe that poor eating habits can cause some of these conditions. Here are some nutritional guidelines you can follow to ensure that you have a well-balanced diet:

- Eat a variety of foods every day to ensure that you are getting all the nutrients that are necessary for the maintenance of good health. These should include fresh fruits and vegetables, fish and fresh seafood, whole grains, nuts, beans and seeds for protein, fibre, minerals and essential fatty acids. Poultry, other meats, butter, eggs and dairy should be eaten in moderation.

- Avoid foods high in cholesterol.

- Limit total fat intake to less than 30% of your calories and keep intake of saturated fats to less than 10%.

- Increase your intake of dietary fibre, such as whole-wheat bread, potatoes, corn, brown rice cooked beans, peas, nuts, seeds, and fresh fruits and leafy vegetables.

- Limit your intake of foods that cause gas. A sudden increase in the consumption of fibre, especially fruits, beans, vegetables and nuts can cause gas, pain and bloating.

- If you have difficulties with dry foods, eat smaller portions, or eat foods that are moist and soft.

- Limit the use of salt and sodium compounds.

- Increase your calcium intake, especially women. (NB: Seniors require at least 1,500mg of calcium per day).

- Avoid too much sugar.

- Drink at least eight (8 ounce) glasses of water per day.

- If you drink alcoholic beverages, do so in moderation.

- Some types of medication can have a negative effect on certain nutrients. If in doubt, seek the advice from your doctor or pharmacist before you take them.

Tips On Adding Variety To Meals

- Forget the view that certain foods should only be eaten at certain times. Try vegetable soup and a tuna fish sandwich on brown bread for breakfast, or a cheese omelette, bran muffin, vegetable salad and fresh fruit for dinner.

- Experiment with recipes created especially for one or two people.

- Combine leftover meats and vegetables into a one-dish casserole that can easily be heated for lunch or dinner, or frozen for later use.

- Share potluck lunches and dinners with friends and acquaintances. Not only will it add variety to your diet, but it is also a great way to make new friends.

Benefits Of Good Nutrition

- Have adequate energy to carry out daily tasks.

- Enjoy good mental health and mental functions/capacities.

- Be resistant to disease.

- Quicker recovery from illnesses, accidents or surgeries.

- Be better able to manage chronic health problems,

which in turn will improve quality of life, mobility and independence.

- Maintain and harmonize system balance.

- Have a more youthful appearance.

EXERCISE

"Active people are biologically younger by as much as 20 or 30 years when they reach the age of 60 or 70 years, compared to people who are inactive and of the same chronological age. " (Martin Katahn, One Meal At A Time.)

Physical Fitness

Physical Fitness is to the human body as fine-tuning is to an engine. It enables us to perform to our potential. Fitness can be described as a condition that helps us to look and feel better, and to do our best. More specifically, it gives us the ability to perform daily tasks vigorously and keeps us in a state of alertness with energy left for enjoying leisure-time activities and meeting emergency demands. It allows one to endure physical demands placed on our body, cope with stress, and deal with different types of situations more effectively. It is the foundation of good health and well-being.

Exercise and Weight Maintenance

Any form of exercise should involve the performance of

the heart, lungs and muscles. Since what we do with our bodies will have a positive impact on our minds, by extension, our level of fitness will definitely have a positive impact on mental alertness and emotional stability. Because exercise also prevents obesity, it helps to protect us from illnesses, which are commonly associated with being overweight.

An important note on the potbelly!

For every inch that your waistline exceeds the size of your chest, you can deduct two years from your life. That is how serious a pot belly is. It means that you are exercising too little, or eating too much, or both.

Apart from facilitating the movement of your trunk and legs, the stomach muscles provide support and protection for the liver, kidneys, pancreas, and stomach. Abdominal muscles that lose their ability to serve as a kind of natural girdle will result in the organs and the lower spine working harder than they were designed to. As a result one can develop digestive disorders and back problems. An estimated 80% of all lower back pain can be traced to a lack of abdominal strength.

Sitting not only gives the stomach muscles very little to do, but also the rest of the body. As a result, in the case of the former, the stomach walls are weakened; and in the case of the latter, we get fat. The combination is devastating and a vicious cycle develops. An increasing waistline makes movement more difficult, hence movement becomes less likely. Less movement means fewer calories are burned and fewer calories burned means that more calories are stored in the body - especially around the middle. It is therefore important that we do some form of exercise to strengthen the abdominal muscles.

Although being overweight is usually commonest cause of a 'spare tyre' around the middle, abdominal prolapse can develop in anyone who neglects to maintain proper posture and sufficient abdominal strength through exercise. Osteoporosis can also cause pot bellies in the slimmest and fittest of persons.

In addition to the prevention of pot belly and its adverse effects on health, the following are some more specific benefits of exercise:

Safety Procedures

It is never too late to reap the benefits of exercise. A regular exercise-training programme can improve fitness and quality of life. It is important that you consult your doctor before you begin any physical activity/exercise programme. Also, if it is possible, use a physiotherapist or an exercise instructor who can give you guidance and supervision to help you maximize the benefits and to avoid injury.

The following are some safety procedures that you

should adopt if you plan to exercise.

- Older people should spend additional time warming up and cooling down.

- They should drink water approximately 15 minutes (before) if they plan to be active for more than 30 minutes.

- All exercise clothing should be loose-fitting to allow for freedom of movement.

- Never wear rubberized or plastic clothing. Such garments interfere with the evaporation of perspiration and cause body temperature to rise to dangerous levels.

- Exercising too hard or too long can cause injuries, such as stress factures, torn ligaments, or pulled muscles. However if you pay attention to the little pains in your body, you can prevent serious injuries.

- The incidence of heat stroke and heat exhaustion as a result of exercising are not common. But you can avoid them by drinking plenty of water and by wearing appropriate clothing. You can also exercise indoors or during cooler times of the day.

- Heart problems may occur in people who exercise too strenuously for their physical condition. Some warning signs are chest pains, extreme breathlessness, light-headedness, or fainting. If you experience any of these symptoms, you should contact your healthcare provider/doctor immediately.

- If you have not been active, you should gradually increase the time you spend exercising. It might be easier to start with a programme of moderate strength training and stretching. Once confidence, strength and balance have improved, you can add cardiovascular exercise. Remember, if you experience chest pains or any other unusual symptom; contact your health care provider immediately.

Your Target Heart Rate

Your maximum heart rate is usually 220 minus your age. However, the figures below are averages and should only be used as a guideline.

Age	Maximum Heart Rate Beats per minute (220 minus your age)	Target Zone 60%	Target Zone 75%
50	170	102	127
55	165	99	123
60	160	96	120
65	155	93	116
70	150	90	113

To calculate your heart rate, find your radial pulse by putting the first and second finger of your right hand on the radial artery of the inner wrist of your left hand, or over the blood vessel on your neck, just to the left of the Adam's apple. Count the number of beats in 30 seconds and multiply by 2. Take your pulse 5 minutes into your exercise routine and again just before ending.

Benefits - Physiological Benefits and Physiological

Physiological Benefits

- *Lowers "bad" cholesterol levels.* This is the type of cholesterol that clogs the arteries and causes heart attacks.

- *Increases "good" cholesterol levels.* "Good" cholesterol protects against heart disease as it keeps the arteries clean.

- *Lowers blood pressure.*

- *Decreases the risk of certain illnesses and death caused by heart disease.*

- *Protects against certain types of cancer*, especially of the breast, digestive tract, and female reproductive organs.

- *Cardiorespiratory endurance.* This enhances the delivery of oxygen and nutrients to the tissues, and the removal of waste from the body.

- *Muscular strength.* Muscles are better able to exert

force for a short period of time.

- *Muscular endurance*. Muscles are better able to sustain repeated contractions and to continue to apply force against fixed objects.

- *Flexibility*. It will result in a better and more extensive range of motion of joints (makes movement easier) and muscles and improves balance.

- *Body composition*. The right types of exercise will help you decrease body fat and increase or maintain muscle mass, thus prevents bone loss.

- *Reduces arthritis pain.*

- *Reduces the risk of injury and muscle pain.*

Psychological Benefits

- Builds self-esteem

- Increases mental alertness

- Contributes to feelings of well-being and euphoria as a result of the production of endorphins.

Prolonged or sustained physical activity (especially aerobic exercise lasting 20 minutes or more) will produce these positive health benefits. Aerobic exercise involves the use of oxygen and in order to maximize the benefits, it must be vigorous and sustained level for at least three times a week. Aerobic-type exercises that are safe for older people include walking, swimming, bicycling and any type of rhythmic exercise performed at a moderate pace. They can get some form of workout by climbing the stairs (at home), rising from a chair, pushing a vacuum cleaner, or broom and carrying groceries.

During exercise it is important to measure your heart rate. Any exercise that does not raise your heart rate to a certain level and keep it there for 20 minutes will not contribute significantly to cardiovascular fitness.

The heart rate you should maintain is called your target heart rate. If you are in good health, you need to set a target zone for the heartbeat, which is determined by your age. Your target zone should be 60% to 75% of your maximum heart rate.

MANAGING STRESS

The elderly face common stresses in the latter part of their lives that can sometimes lead to behavioural problems. High levels of stress are associated with greater difficulties in falling asleep. This can result in the body becoming more vulnerable to illnesses.

General Stressors

- Death of a spouse.

- Physical illnesses, especially chronic illness that raises issues of dependence versus independence.

- Social isolation, accompanied by feelings of loneliness.

- Coping with ageing.

- Financial insecurities.

Assisting The Elderly To Cope With Stress

- It is important that you plan ahead. Put aside money for your future.

- Get involved in some form of social activity. For example, playing cards, bingo and singing, or join a social club.

- Get involved in an exercise programme. It is important that you keep active, as you get older.

- Get connected to your spiritual side.

PREVENTING DEPRESSION

Depression is in the background as a causative factor or a coexisting condition in most of the diseases (such as heart attack and stroke) facing the elderly over age 50 years.

What Is Depression

Depression is a serious health problem that affects the

total person. It is more than the 'blues' or 'blahs', or the normal everyday ups and downs. In fact, when that 'down' mood, along with other symptoms lasts for more than a couple of weeks, the condition may be clinical depression. In addition to the feelings, it can result in a change in behaviour, physical health and appearance, and the ability to handle everyday decisions and pressures.

Causes Of Depression

Although scientists do not yet know all the causes of depression, there seems to be biological and emotional factors that may increase the likelihood that an individual will develop a depressive disorder. Research over the past decade strongly suggests a genetic link to depressive disorders, that is, depression can run in families. In addition the elder can experience depression as a result of:

- Bad life experiences, such as debilitating illnesses.

- Side effects of some medication.

- Certain personality patterns, such as difficulty handling stress.

- Financial difficulties

- Loss of contact with family members or friends.

- Extreme pessimism about the future.

- Low self-esteem

- Abuse

- Neglect

Symptoms Of Depression

It is important to note that it is often difficult for the person who is depressed to think clearly or recognize his or her own symptoms. They may therefore need your help. The following are some symptoms of depression:

- Expressions or feelings of sadness, emptiness, hopelessness, pessimism, guilt, helplessness or worthlessness.

- Negative thinking, such as expressions of suicide.

- Inability to make decisions.

- Inability to concentrate and remember.

- Loss of interest or pleasure in things/activities that they once enjoyed.

- Sudden change in behaviour. They are restless or more irritable, or they want to be alone.

- Heavy consumption of alcohol or drugs, or smoking heavily.

Treatment

Depression can be treated. Even the most severe cases

can be helped. Symptoms can be relieved quickly with psychological therapies, such as talk therapy and medication. Not only does treatment lessen the severity, it may also reduce the duration or length of time and may prevent recurrence or additional bouts of depression.

There are many places in the community where people with depressive disorders can be diagnosed and treated. Help is available from:

- A family doctor
- Religious leader, such as a pastor or priest
- Mental health specialist
- Private clinics
- Other health professionals

In addition you can:

- Talk to a close friend
- Re-establish your connection with family members and friends
- Get connected to your spiritual side

MAINTAINING FAMILY TIES

The family, (as well as friends) is as important in later life as during childhood. It is an important support group that creates joy and a sense of belonging through time spent together and expressions of love and affection. Time spent with family members and expressions of love become even more important as the elderly adjust to the major changes in their lives.

Ways In Which You Can Maintain Family Contact

- Visiting family members or friends

- Inviting family members or friends to visit you.

- Writing letters

- Use the technology that is currently available. For example, the telephone, cellular phones, and computer.

- Going on holidays or picnics with members of your family or friends

The methods of maintaining contact with both family members and friends are not limited to the above. There are many other ways in which this can be done. You can devise creative ways of doing so, and be sure to enjoy the experience.

SAFETY

The elderly are often at risk of many hazards as sometimes they are unable to help themselves. Family members or care-givers need to assist the elderly to ensure that:

- The home is safe from intruders.

- They do not wear too much jewelry in public.

- They do not travel with too much money on their person.

- They do not open their homes to strangers

- The home is built free of known hazards that can result in falls.

Tips For Elderly Drivers

The Elderly Driver

Growing older is not necessarily accompanied by loss of interest in driving. However, you should only do so if you are visually and physically capable, as the possession of a driver's licence does not mean that you are able to or should drive. For your safety and the safety of others, (as you get older) you will need to pay special attention to the following age-related changes that may affect you ability to drive:

- Increased sensitivity to light or glare.

- Slower adjustment to the dark

- Diminished coordination

- Slower reaction time

- Changes in your hearing and eyesight and other sensory impairment

- Illness that can result in fender-benders or serious accidents

Compensating For Your Limitations

- *Change your driving habits.* If you feel uneasy on the road, think about how, when and where you drive. Try driving fewer miles, less often and slower. Plan trips carefully by choosing the route to be taken beforehand and drive less at night and during rush hours.

- *Wear your seatbelt.* Older drivers are more likely to be injured or killed in an accident than younger, as the former tend to have bones that are more fragile. This reduces the ability to withstand the trauma of an accident. Safety belts distribute the full force of the impact across the strongest parts of your body, help to prevent you from hitting the steering wheel, the windows or the dashboard and help to keep you from being thrown from the vehicle. You should ensure that the belt is securely fastened and properly positioned over the shoulder, across the chest, and low on the stomach.

- *Check your eyesight and hearing.* Over one-third of all older people experience hearing loss. This makes it more difficult to hear in busy traffic. Other types of visual problems may also develop. For example:

o You may become more sensitive to glare and adapt slower to darkness.

o You may have more difficulty adjusting your focus from distant objects to near ones and vice-versa.

o You may need more light.

o Your reaction time may be slower.

o Your peripheral vision may diminish.

o Your ability to quickly and accurately distinguish colours may diminish.

Visual Driving Tips

- Wear proper eyeglasses for day and night driving (you may need two different types).

- Do not wear sunglasses or tinted lenses when driving at night.

- Wear good quality sunglasses in sunlight.

- Keep glasses clean.

- Avoid frames with wide sidepieces as they block side vision.

- Look at the big picture when driving. Be constantly aware of your surroundings. Watch the road ahead and check either side for vehicles, children, animals or hazards. Glance frequently in the rearview mirror and at the instrument panel.

- Avoid driving at dusk, sunset or at night.

- Keep pace with traffic flow.

- Keep headlights properly adjusted.

- Keep headlights, taillights windshields clean, and side windows clean.

Tips For Pedestrians

As pedestrians (those who walk on the streets), the onus is on you to protect yourselves. Here are some tips.

- Always face the oncoming vehicle when walking on the road.

- Walk on sidewalks (if provided).

- Obey all road signals.

- Use pedestrian crossings when crossing the road. If there is no pedestrian crossing, *'look left, then right, and left again'*, then walk across the road.

- Always give the oncoming vehicle enough time to stop, or that it comes to a complete stop before you attempt to cross the road.

- Try and make eye contact with the driver of the oncoming vehicle. After he/she acknowledges that he/she sees you, walk across the road.

- If you have visual, hearing or any physical problems, ask someone to assist you.

Driving And Prescription Drugs

Some prescription and over-the-counter medication can affect your vision while driving. These include prescription cold and sinus remedies, sleeping pills, tranquilizers, sedatives, painkillers and prescription drugs for any condition. Even aspirin, when used extensively, can adversely affect vision. Whatever the drug, know its side effect before getting behind the wheel.

Public Transportation

At some point you may need to use the public transportation system. The following are some safety tips you should practise:

- Have fare ready to prevent losing your balance while looking for change.

- Remain alert and brace yourself when the bus is coming to a stop or turning a corner.

- Do not carry too many packages. Leave one hand free to grasp railings.

- Do not display large amounts of cash while in a public transport.

Making The Environment Safe For The Elderly

As we get older, it is important that we make our environment safer. In some cases, we have to modify our environment to accommodate the changing conditions that are associated with ageing.

The following are some environmental threats to the elderly:

- Poor sanitation
- Poor food storage
- Wet floors
- Uneven sidewalks
- Improper public facilities, such as rails and lighting

Here are some tips for making the environment safer for the elderly

- Use bright and direct lighting in all areas of the home and public facilities.
- Reduce the risks of falling by eliminating tripping hazards, such as throw rugs and cushions.

- Put in full-length railings on both sides of stairways.

- Put light switches at both ends of stairways.

- Lower cabinet height to minimize the need to reach.

- Use straight-back chairs with arms and hard seats, whether at the end of the dining table or in the living room. These are easier to get out of than soft seats.

Preventing Falls

Falls are the commonest accidental injury among the elderly. Here are some tips to help prevent falls.

- Ensure that the floor and carpets are in good condition and secured firmly to the floor. Loose rugs and "snags" are falls waiting to happen. Kitchen floors should be made of non-slip material.

- Stairs should be well lit and a light switch should be placed at both ends of the stairs. Each step should have a non-skid tread. Make sure the banister is strong.

- Night lights should be placed in areas such as bathrooms or kitchens where an older person is likely to walk at night. At other times each room should be well lit.

- Telephones should be conveniently positioned so

that no one has to rush or stumble over furniture to answer the phone. Also telephone cords and electric wires should be securely fastened.

- Railings should be installed in bathtubs and, if necessary, beside the toilet.

- Use a non-skid bath mat or have a non-slip surface installed in the tub or on the floor. Put a seat in the tub.

- Limit the use of low chairs or on furniture that are on casters.

- Try to control the activity of pets to avoid tripping.

- Have smoke alarms installed throughout the home.

- Wear shoes that fit properly and that have low heels. Do not walk around in socks or stockings that will make you slip.

- Avoid the use of extension cords. If you use them, ensure that they are securely fastened.

- Use a sturdy step stool when reaching for objects in high places or put items in places where they can be easily reached.

- Get proper training in the use of a cane or a walker, as improper use may lead to falls. Ensure that it is adjusted to your height and use it appropriately.

General Safety Tips

- If you are taking medication that lowers blood pressure, ensure that you take them in between meals to avoid a significant drop in blood sugar. If you become dizzy after meals, eat smaller portions.

- Take prescribed medication as ordered. In addition, be careful of medication that makes you drowsy.

- Have eyes and ears examined annually or regularly.

- Get involved in some type of exercise programme that will improve strength, gait and mobility.

- Ensure that hot and cold faucets in the bathroom and kitchen are clearly marked.

- Ensure that the controls for the stove are clearly marked.

- Install smoke alarms throughout the home.

- Ensure that naked lights (kerosine lamps) are kept away from flamable material.

Be extremely careful, especially if you are experiencing dizzy or fainting spell and weakness. If there you have problems with vision or coordination, your risks of falling are increased. If you are on medication, ensure that you know the side effects (if there are any). For example, many blood pressure medications can cause drowsiness and depression.

Maintaining A Proper Posture

As we get older, it becomes more and more important to be attentive to our posture. Age causes some changes in the discs that separate our spine vertebrae. We lose a little height as these discs become a bit thinner with age. This causes other soft tissues like ligaments and muscles to become a little less tense than when we were younger. This slight reduction in tension can cause an increase in that 'rounded over/shoulder' posture we get. So it is even more important as we age that we sit and stand tall.

Strengthening the muscles that squeeze the shoulder blades together is very important in reducing round-shouldered posture. In turn, reducing round-shouldered posture is very important in keeping the shoulder joints correctly aligned for maximum functional shoulder use.

Sitting and standing tall with shoulder blades gently squeezed together also improved the ability of the lungs to expand more fully when you breathe in. Increased intake of oxygen provides an opportunity for more oxygen to get to the brain and muscles, thereby helping our mental alertness and muscle strength, to maintain a higher activity level.

In addition to sitting and standing tall and keeping the shoulder blades gently squeezed together, it is important to keep the head gently tucked and eyes looking ahead to assist in the prevention of headaches, neck strain and pain.

MAINTAINING A HEALTHY ENVIRONMENT

The environment refers to the combination of external or extrinsic physical conditions that affect and influence our growth and development. It also refers to the complex social and cultural conditions, which affect the nature of an individual or community. In this regard, therefore, our environment can greatly influence our health. As senior citizens, you can do a lot about your personal environment - physical surroundings, health habits and practices- to extend your life and improve fitness and appearance. In other words, an improvement in your physical and personal environment can have a positive impact on your health.

Personal Hygiene

This refers to the conditions and practices that serve to promote or preserve health and well-being.

- You should have a bath/shower, comb your hair at least once per day; and brush your teeth at least three times per day, or after every meal.

- When you sneeze, handle meat or other raw poultry, go to the bathroom, etc. you should wash your hands and the environs (such as your cutting board in the kitchen). This is the most important thing you can do to prevent the spread of germs and infections. In many instances, it is the most important preventive measure you can take.

- You should have at least five or more servings of fruits per day. This will help keep the doctor, with some forms of cancer and other disorders away. A well-nourished body will be able to withstand the ravishes of the environment than one that is not properly nourished.

- If you smoke, contact your health care provider who can assist you to quit.

- Ensure that your surroundings are clean, well ventilated and have adequate natural or artificial light.

- Regular and safe supply of potable and palatable water for all personal and household uses should be identified and used.

- You should ensure that you have suitable living arrangements.

Garbage Disposal

The ways in which garbage is handled, stored or disposed of can affect our health and well-being. It is therefore important that you devise safe and sanitary methods of disposing garbage, sewage and other wastes that are generated from your daily activities.

In addition to the above, you should:
- Clean up and dispose of food scraps instantly.

- Empty household rubbish daily and keep outside and inside bins tightly closed.

- Put scraps outside for birds on tables or in feeders.

- Do not burn garbage, either bury or recycle it.

- Wash your hands with soap and water (for at least fifteen seconds) after you have handled garbage.

Spring Cleaning

This refers to an extensive cleaning of the home. It is a tedious but important task, as over the years we have collected a lot of personal items, equipment, among other things that clutter our personal space. We should therefore try to get rid of the things that we no longer use. A good indication to determine what goes and what stays is frequency of use. That is, if you have not used it in the past six months to a year, you will probably not use it again. These items can be donated to charity, and remember, *'one man's junk is another man's treasure'*.

EXTEND YOUR LIFE BY YOUR LIFESTYLE

"To know how to grow old is the master work of wisdom, and one of the most difficult chapters in the great art of living." (Henri Frederic Amiel, 1821-1881)

As far as science is concerned, the methods for extending our lifespan will be found in genetic engineering and we have not yet discovered the secrets. It helps to be born into a family where people live a long life. And, of course, it also is important that we protect ourselves from diseases, poisonous substances and the risk of fatal accidents. In addition, there are different philosophies, based on human wisdom and anecdotal evidence, which suggest numerous other means of prolonging life.

Lifestyle Extension Tips

In addition to ensuring proper nutrition and frequent exercise, here are some suggestions, which may be helpful:

- Drink alcohol in moderation. Heavy drinking decreases one's lifespan by many years.

- Do not use illicit drugs.

- Stop smoking. Smoking two packs of cigarettes per day takes seven years from your life span.

- Maintain your weight at a healthy level. Research has confirmed that almost every healthy person who lives for a relatively long time is slim. Very few have been overweight. Diets that cause you to lose weight only to gain it back are not considered healthy. The way to lose weight is to exercise and gradually cut back on fats, sugars and too much food.

- Get a good night's sleep. If you cannot sleep, try to find a method of relaxation that works for you. It may also help if you increase your exercise time or get involved in interesting activities.

- Ignore your chronological age. Age is not the number of your birthdays. It is an attitude, an awareness, a feeling. So keep active and maintain a youthful attitude. As the old saying goes, *'you are as old as you feel'*.

- Learn to relax. Here are some suggestions:

  o Deliberately slow the pace of your life.

  o Live fully in the present moment.

  o Do only one thing at a time

  o Do not be afraid to say "no." Say 'NO' to demands on your time that cause stress.

  o Learn to accept the fact that if you cannot complete a job today it is acceptable to finish it later.

  o Spend some quality time with yourself everyday.

  o Enjoy life to the fullest. Learn to see, smell, touch and feel everything around you right now.

- Develop a powerful will to live, and never give up.

What most distinguishes some older persons (from the rest) is their indestructible capacity to rebound from misfortune and adversity.

- Make important and achievable goals. As soon as you achieve one goal, immediately move on to another. Choose only goals that are realistic and achievable, otherwise you are defining dreams and are likely to fail or become frustrated.

- Create a newer and stronger image. Think about your strengths and forget or work on your weaknesses. Walk tall and erect with a quick step. Allow yourself to feel optimistic and confident about the future. Adopt a positive mental attitude and feel good about yourself

- Be a success. Success is an essential component in creating a powerful will to live. We can readily experience the exuberance of success by making a list of small successes, each of which can be attained in 15 minutes, like cleaning a bicycle or the interior of your car. Achieving several small successes can fortify your will to live and make it easier to attain more important goals that can leave you flushed with the inspiration of success.

- Minimize stress in your life. Most stress is due to change, so expose yourself to as little change as possible. Live a systematic life that is in harmony with the rhythms of the nature. However, it is sometimes just as stressful to resist change in an ever changing world. In such instances, it is best to somewhat alter your perspective and overcome your fears.

- Have a positive mental attitude. Fear, anxiety and worry are deadly killers and make us more suscep-tible to illness. For instance, researchers have found a link between susceptibility to the common cold and state of mind. A person who is depressed is more likely to catch a cold than his/her (happier) counter-part. Similarly, people who hold on to hostility or anger are five times more likely to develop cardio-vascular disease than those who do not. Although we are not yet fully able to understand the reason for all of this, it is clear, that our attitudes greatly influ-ence our health. It therefore pays to adopt an attitude that is free from anger, resentment and negativism.

- Live happily. Laugh a lot. Researchers have shown that fun and laughter have therapeutic benefits, espe-cially in the promotion of health and longevity. Those who live longer lives do not take themselves seriously. They often laugh at themselves and their mistakes. They approach each new and different experience with an enthusiastic attitude, and possess an almost childlike enthusiasm for spontaneous fun or play.

- Be a loving and generous person. Dr. Solomonovich, a Russian gerontologist, spent sometime living in close proximity with the Abkhasian people. He reported that he never heard them utter a harsh word. Other researchers who have studied groups of people that have a long lifespan have also observed that these people are invariably generous, loving and unselfish.

- Avoid living alone. People live healthier and longer lives when they have close and loving relationships. Studies from around the world have shown that loneliness impacts negatively on health and life. Human beings are by nature 'social beings' and thrive best when there is companionship. Gerontologists agree that we can extend life significantly by creating a compatible and stable relationship with family members, friends and by being actively involved in a number of social organizations.

- Maintain a monogamous sexual relationship. It has been reported that regular sexual activity with one permanent partner increases life expectancy by at least two years. Almost all healthy individuals and those who live longer lives stayed married and enjoyed regular lovemaking.

- Keep growing. People who live longer lives are

independent and adventurous. They maintain a balance between being afraid and taking occasional risks, which do not endanger their well-being. We become old on the day that we stop growing. Ensure that you do not fall out of the mainstream of life, thoughts and ideas by seeking safety in the status quo. Numerous studies have shown that ceasing to grow is synonymous with physical atrophy and mental withdrawal.

- Stay mentally active throughout life. A series of studies show that an active mind is man's greatest weapon against ageing. People live longer when they use their brain to acquire and practise wisdom. Although the brain ages slower than any other organ, without constant use it can deteriorate and our memory will start to fade.

- Believe in and rely on a higher power. Researchers have shown that all forms of spiritual belief and faith have a powerful and positive effect on health and longevity. It can be inferred from these studies that your faith can help you to better deal with stressful situations. Therefore you are able to relax and enjoy living.

- Continue to work at a satisfying job for as long as possible. Work makes us who and what we are. Work is life and life is work. Being without a job can be harmful to your well-being, as it is usually difficult to maintain a healthy lifestyle if you are not involved in some type of work. Most people, who retire at the age of 65, die within a few months unless they become involved in meaningful hobbies, volunteer work or their occupation.

Types Of Work Environments That Optimize Our Health

Scientists, who have studied the effects that different types of occupation have on our health, have concluded that we will enjoy optimum health and longevity, if we work in an environment:

- In which we are free to make all or most of our decisions. We should be under no one's authority or supervision. The closer we are to being our own boss, the better it is.

- That allows us to make maximum use of our abilities, skills and talents. An underutilized person is invariably frustrated.

- Where there is scope for promotion. That is, it allows us to reach a position of eminence in our chosen field.

- In which we can work at our own pace, free from all deadlines and pressures.

- In which successful work leaves no stress scars.

Enjoyable and satisfying work is synonymous with play.

- That allows us to do our very best work and to take pride in the work we do. It should encourage us to aim for higher goals and prepare us to tackle challenging new tasks, which will develop a feeling of success and accomplishment.

- In which we are able to work without any pressure to retire for as long as necessary.

Spiritual Health

At this stage of life, it is expected that the individuals would have achieved or fulfilled most of their basic needs. However, the need for spiritual fulfillment is highest at this point. In a research done in the United States, it was reported that elderly persons who attend church regularly, or are involved in some form of spiritual practice tend to live longer than their counterpart.

It is therefore important that family members and significant others support the elderly at this time. They should be encouraged to become a part of a group that fosters spiritual growth and development.

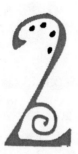

What you should know about your

MEDICAL CARE

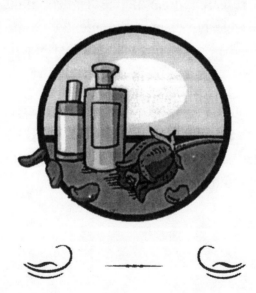

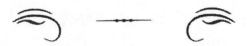

HEALTH

Regardless of age, each of us should have a personal doctor. This doctor, also referred to as a primary care physician, is in essence the gatekeeper of your health. In addition to being available for you, his or her duties are:

- *To establish a plan of preventive care.* As the saying goes, 'a stitch in time saves nine' and the whole idea behind preventive care is to catch and mend any 'rip that may appear in the fabric of your health' before it results in the loss of a seam. This is done through regular check-ups and screening tests.

- *The management of chronic conditions.* Until very recently, "acute" illnesses such as influenza, diphtheria and tuberculosis were the primary causes of death. As we approach the 21st century, some of our main enemies are the chronic diseases that work slowly over time and eventually become debilitating. These include hypertension, heart disease, arthritis and diabetes. One of the primary functions of your doctor is to prevent or control these conditions as best as possible, so that in the case of the former they either do not develop or in the case of the latter they do the least harm.

- *Patient education.* When it comes to your health, what you do not know can and does harm you. Your doctor is there to educate you about staying healthy and counsel you when you become ill.

- *Referrals to other doctors.* Sometimes your doctor may need to consult someone else, such as a specialist, when he is faced with a problem that goes beyond his area of expertise. For example, if you have a heart problem, he or she may send you to see a cardiologist who deals exclusively with heart problems. Your personal physician should not only tell you when you should see a specialist but should be able to refer you to the best, since most doctors know the quality physicians in the community, as well as the ones to avoid. In addition, if you are being treated by a specialist, your doctor should do follow-up checks to ensure that things are going as planned.

- *Support.* Sometimes you may need someone who can soothe your fears and tell you that it is going to be all right. An important role that your doctor plays is to simply be there if you have a question or need a helping hand.

- *Advocacy*. The world of health care is like a jungle for many seniors. Insurance companies and hospitals sometimes make it harder rather than easier to get quality health care. In such cases, you should be able to rely on your doctor to step in and take charge of the situation, whether it is for prolonged hospitalization or additional medical care.

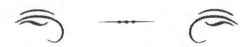

PREVENTIVE CARE

The best thing you can do to protect yourself and your health is not to get sick in the first place or, at the very least, become aware of the problems while they are still treatable. This proactive approach to health care is called "preventive care." The following can be done to protect your health and well-being:

- *Educate yourself.* The first step of preventive care is educating yourself about your body and its needs. Many organizations for seniors have educational booklets that cover every subject, from nutrition, exercise to the warning signs of all diseases. In addition to booklets, senior citizens' centres offer educational opportunities. Your doctor can also provide you with educational materials to assist you.

The preventive practices outlined below are provided by the Jamaican Heart Association, the Cancer Society and other experts in the field. They are guidelines and may not apply to your individual case. Your specific needs may be different and your doctor may recommend additional tests not listed here.

- *Immunizations.* Decide with your doctor whether or not you need yearly flu shots or any other inoculation.

- *History.* Your health history, which is important to a successful diagnosis, should be updated every two and a half years after the age of 61 years and annually after the age of 75 years.

- *Mammogram.* A mammogram is an x-ray photograph or radiograph of the breast. It identifies cancer too small to locate manually. This test is recommended once between the ages of 35 and 40 to get a baseline and then every two years until age 50. Thereafter, an annual test is recommended. Self-examination of the breast for lumps is recommended on a monthly basis.

- *Stool Slide Tests.* This is an analysis of the stool to search for hidden traces of blood, the appearance of which could mean cancer or some other disorder in the digestive tract. Stool slide tests are recommended once a year for everyone over the age of 50 years.

- *Sigmoidoscopies.* A sigmoidoscopy is a procedure that allows the physician to see within the colon with the aid of a flexible tube. While the test is uncomfortable, it provides valuable information, as it can detect cancerous cells at a very early stage when it is easier to treat. It is recommended that both men and women do this test every three years after two normal exams one year apart, starting at the age of 50 years.

- *Urinalysis.* The urine is like a road map that details the workings of many vital organs. It is recommended that a urinalysis be done every year after the age of 40 years.

- *Blood Tests.* Like the urine, the blood is a window to the workings of the body. Blood tests should be taken every five years until age 60 years and every two and a half years thereafter, if good results have been documented.

- *Blood Pressure.* A healthy person who shows no signs of high blood pressure or heart disease, should do blood pressure checks every two and a half to five years until age 61, and every two and a half years until age 75 years, after which it should be taken annually.

- *Pelvic Exams.* All healthy women over the age of 40 should do a pelvic exam once per year.

- *ECGs.* Baseline ECG tests are usually recommended at ages 20, 40 and 60.

- *Physical exams.* Physical exams and the rate at which they are done vary, and often depend on what your physician is looking for. A thorough heart and vascular system checkup should be done every five years until age 50 years, every two and a half years until age 75 years, and annually thereafter.

- *Accident Prevention.* When an elderly person is hospitalized because of an accident, the stay is usually longer and recovery time slower than that of a younger person. As a result, all senior citizens should practise safety rules. Ensure that the home is as free as possible of safety hazards. (See making the environment safe for the elderly).

The Jamaican Cancer Society also recommends an examination for cancers of the thyroid, testicles, prostate, ovaries, lymph nodes and skin every three years until age 40. Thereafter, it is recommended that you be screened every year for cancer.

All these preventive procedures are important, but what if you do not have the money to pay for them? Since many traditional insurance policies do not cover preventive care, this could be a problem. You should therefore work with your doctor to get as much assistance for screening as possible. Your doctor can "diagnose" most conditions that would require screening. You should also work out a schedule of payment with your doctor.

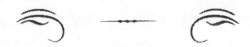

DISEASES THAT AFFECT THE ELDERLY
- DESCRIPTION, SYMPTOMS AND PROGNOSIS

Each stage of our life is made up of joys, sorrows, pains and afflictions. However, certain physical and medical conditions/challenges are more common in older people than in younger people. The senior citizens, who are educated about these conditions and have a proactive approach as it relates to their health and well-being, will recognize the symptoms immediately and deal with them accordingly.

ALZHEIMER'S DISEASE

Description: Alzheimer's Disease is an insidious form of dementia caused by the deterioration of brain cells.

Symptoms: Alzheimer's disease is characterized by one's inability to remember recent events or difficulty performing familiar tasks. As the disease progresses, the victim may undergo severe changes in personality and have difficulty remembering family members. Ultimately, the victim is unable to care for him or herself.

Not all memory problems or similar difficulties are symptomatic of Alzheimer's disease.

Prognosis: Unfortunately, not good. Alzheimer's is a debilitating disease with no known cure. Also, there is no treatment currently available to stop or slow the progression of the disease. If you or a loved one has been diagnosed by a competent physician and have obtained a second opinion that the problems are a result of Alzheimer s (there is no 100% diagnosis except during an autopsy), you should:

o *Get another opinion.* You should consult a neurologist and/or a geriatric psychologist to triple check the diagnosis. Severe depression has, on occasion, been misdiagnosed as Alzheimer's.

o *Adjust your life.* If the diagnosis is confirmed, the victim should make adjustments so as to maximize his or her potential. For example, victims should start to record events to make up for memory loss. Another tip is to develop the habit of leaving important items such as glasses, dentures, pocket books and the other personal items in the same place where they can be easily found. Also, victims and families must be patient and be willing to accept help.

o *Plan ahead.* Since the disease progresses slowly, those who have been diagnosed sometimes have time to make plans concerning their care and estate. Areas to deal with include retirement, legal affairs, support services, living arrangements and medical care.

ARTHRITIS

Description: Arthritis has a crippling effect on most senior citizens. Depending on its severity, arthritis can turn everyday activities, such as getting out of bed into an excruciating task.

Symptoms: The most common type is degenerative arthritis. Victims of this condition, experience pains in the joints of the hands, knees, hips and feet. They may also experience muscle and back pain. Persons who have systemic arthritis, such as rheumatoid arthritis, may also experience weight loss and fever.

Prognosis: Your primary health care physician can treat the pain in most cases. In other cases, the victims may need to see a specialist, such as a rheumatologist or an orthopaedist. Doctors can prescribe pain medication, beginning with simple aspirin, and can also give medication to reduce swelling. Proper exercise or prescribed therapy can also help. In a few cases, a badly damaged joint, such as the hip can be surgically replaced.

BLURRED VISION OR LOSS OF SIGHT

Description: Many senior citizens experience difficulty with their sight. They can experience such a problem as farsightedness, which can be corrected with reading glasses to more severe problems, such as glaucoma and cataracts, which can lead to blindness.

Symptoms: Anything that reduces vision or one's ability to read, such as 'haziness' in the vision or "rainbow rings" around the eyes. There may be no symptoms, especially with glaucoma; so regular eye checkups are necessary.

Prognosis: A new pair of glasses or eye drops. For more serious problems, surgery may be recommended. Early detection is vital in the treatment of serious eye problems.

CANCER

Description: Cancer is an insidious disease that comes in many sizes, shapes and forms. It can present itself as a tumour, as in the case of colon and breast cancer, as a skin lesion or as a condition of the blood, known as leukemia. It can be fatal. However, in many cases, it can be cured if detected early.

Symptoms: There are too many types of cancers with different types of symptoms to list all in this publication. However, you should familiarize yourself with the "The Seven Deadly Signs of Cancer" as outlined by the Cancer Society:

- Change in bowel or bladder habits.
- A sore that does not heal.
- Unusual bleeding or discharge.
- Thickening of or lump in breast (or elsewhere).
- Indigestion or difficulty in swallowing.
- Obvious change in wart or mole.
- Nagging cough or hoarseness.

Prognosis: Cancer treatments include chemotherapy, radiation and surgery or a combination of two or all three. Many believe that the patient's attitude is also important. Regardless of the method of treatment pursued, early detection is definitely important to a successful outcome. Prevention is also the only cure. You should also consult with your doctor if you experience two or more of the above signs, or if you have any doubts as to your status.

DIABETES

Description: Diabetes is a disease of the pancreas that prevents it from producing enough insulin to convert food into energy. As a result, glucose (blood sugar) cannot enter cells, so it builds up in the blood. Diabetes can lead to blindness, loss of limbs and death. There are two types of diabetes, "insulin dependent" also referred to as "juvenile onset" and "non-insulin dependent" which affects many seniors.

Symptoms: The most common early symptoms are increased thirst and frequent urination. Other symptoms include increased appetite, infections of the skin or urinary tract, slow healing of cuts and bruises, lack of energy, pain or numbness in the legs or feet and blurred vision. Non-insulin dependent or "mature onset" diabetes may have little or no symptom at all.

Prognosis: There is no known cure for diabetes, but

it can be controlled. It is important that you watch your diet by eating less sugar and fat and eating more carbohydrates and fibre. In some cases, diet alone is not sufficient to manage this condition, your doctor may then prescribe oral medication or insulin injections. All victims must monitor their conditions closely. For more details contact your local chapter of the Jamaican Diabetes Association or consult your doctor.

HEARING LOSS

Description: Approximately 50 % of seniors up to age 79 years experience some form of hearing loss. This can be temporary or permanent, and may be as a result of a side effect of a medication. Many people do not report hearing loss to their doctor, which is to their disadvantage, as most types of hearing impairments can be easily treated.

Symptoms: Hearing loss has fairly obvious symptoms. Words become difficult to understand, normal conversational tones sound muffled, the victim starts to speak loudly and often asks others to repeat themselves. Hearing loss may also make an older person appear to be confused, unintelligent or uncooperative, which can in turn lead to depression and withdrawal.

Prognosis: Often surgery or hearing aid will correct the problem, or in most cases, simply flushing the ear of accumulated wax is all that is necessary.

HEART DISEASE AND HEART ATTACKS

Description: There are many types of heart disease. The most common type is a disease of the arteries called arteriosclerosis, better known as hardening of the arteries. This condition is caused by the build-up of plaque in the coronary arteries, which slowly cuts off the blood supply to the heart muscle and in turn leads to a heart attack.

Symptoms: Any pain or feeling of fullness or squeezing in the chest that lasts for more than two minutes should be considered as a possible heart attack. Also, pain in the shoulder or jaw can be a sign of a heart attack. Vomiting and sweating frequently accompany the pain. Older people may also suffer silent symptoms rather than painful ones. In such cases, the person may simply feel breathless or experience a sudden state of confusion or change in mental status, without experiencing any chest pain. In other cases, there are no symptoms and it only reveals itself when an ECG or cholesterol blood count test is done.

Prognosis: There is a lot you can do to prevent heart

disease. Usually a simple diet to reduce cholesterol is the first step. Your doctor should advise you get involved in a regular exercise programme, such as walking or riding a stationary bike. He/she should educate you about heart disease and about the things you can do to avoid or reduce its effects.

HYPERTENSION

Description: Hypertension, also known as high blood pressure, occurs when the blood flows through the system at such high pressure that it causes damage to blood vessels and vital organs, such as the kidneys. It is a major cause of stroke (the bleeding or clotting of a blood vessel of the brain which damages the brain, due to loss of oxygen or other nutrients). One of the more common signs of a stroke is a sudden weakness or numbness often felt in the face, arm, and leg or on one side of the body, which may or may not be temporary. There may also be a slurring of words, loss of speech or unexplained dizziness or falls. Hypertension can also lead to kidney failure and loss of use of other organs.

Prognosis: Hypertension can be controlled by reducing salt in the diet, changing of your diet, losing weight, regular exercise, and if necessary, medication. If medication is necessary, be sure you work closely with your doctor and report all side effects. It is important that you use the right drug and in the correct dosage. For more detailed information about this condition, see your doctor.

INCONTINENCE

Description: Incontinence is the involuntary loss of control over urine, stool or both. The loss can be minor, such as leakage of a small amount of urine upon sneezing (stress incontinence) to a total inability to control elimination functions.

It can be as a result of four (4) reasons:

- o Urological (medical problems in the genito-urinary tract).

- o Neurological (disease of the brain, spine or nerves).

- o Psychological (depression, anxiety)

- o Environmental factors, such as a handicap that prevents access to a bathroom or as a side effect of certain medication.

Symptoms: Full or partial inability to control bladder or bowel functions.

Prognosis: Treatment for incontinence can range from special exercises, medication, and surgery to devices such as catheters. There are also special undergarments that can be worn to protect themselves from embarrassment.

THE "ITS ONLY OLD AGE" SYNDROME

This type of attitude arises from a belief by many doctors and other health care professionals that your health problems are a result of old age.

Symptoms: The most obvious symptom is failure to take your health complaints seriously.

Prognosis: Find a doctor who understands and respects the health needs of older people. Insist on being treated with respect and courtesy. Get a second opinion if necessary, and always be aware of this form of discrimination because it creates unnecessary suffering to thousands, perhaps millions of people.

There are other common problems that senior citizens face, such as impotence, prostate conditions (which tend to affect older men), osteoporosis and depression. The key to dealing with any problem that may arise is to:

o   Find a doctor who cares about you.

o   Get as much information as possible, which
    will assist you to make informed decisions
    about treatment.

o   Develop the attitude that "this will not get me
    down, this too shall pass".

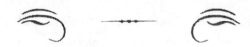

WHAT YOU SHOULD KNOW ABOUT . . .

At some point in our lives we may need to visit the doctor, pharmacist or hospital. As we grow older, it is almost inevitable. In order to gain maximum benefits from these visits, there are important questions that you should ask and procedures that you should follow.

YOUR DOCTOR AND YOU

It is important that you have a personal doctor or a family practitioner. This refers to a doctor who specializes in general family care and has training in paediatrics, general surgery, psychiatry, obstetrics as well as internal medicine. The type of doctor you select is up to you. However, you should ensure that the physician has an interest in geriatrics (the treatment of older people). This is important because your medical needs will change, as you get older.

Regular Checkups

Health becomes a more important issue for people, as they grow older. The little pains and aches that were easily overlooked in younger years, become harder to ignore. There is not as much energy as before. Stamina is not at the level it used to be and there is even more awareness of our dietary indiscretions.

These realizations force us to face the fact that we can no longer take our health for granted. From this point, into the future, our health and quality of life depend on proper self-care, regular preventive check-ups and appropriate medical care or follow-up treatments as required.

At this time, also, visits to the doctor become more frequent and more important. A conventional schedule of health maintenance should proceed as follows.

- A complete physical examination every three to five years (including professional manual breast examination for women and professional testicular and prostate examinations for men.)

- A serum cholesterol test at least every five years, especially if previous tests were high.

- An annual pelvic examination and cervical pap smear for women after the age 40 years.

What To Expect From Your Regular Check-up

When you go for your regular check-up, expect the following tests:

- Vision (performed occasionally, unless specified)
- Hearing (same as above)
- Blood pressure
- Weight
- Temperature (performed occasionally)
- Heart, lungs, and breathing, performed with the aid of a stethoscope
- A blood test for serum glucose cholesterol or others
- A urinalysis
- A breast examination for women
- A manual testicular and prostate examination for men.
- An examination designed to evaluate the state of any specific conditions you have described to your doctor.

What To Do When you Go to The Doctor

Write down any health related questions that you have before your appointment. In addition, you can ask these general questions:

    o **Do you visit nursing homes?** At some point

in many seniors' lives a stay at a nursing home may become necessary. Most stays are not permanent, but whether or not it is, you should keep your personal physician. If your doctor does not visit homes, then he or she is simply not able to give you the care that is necessary. The time to find this out is before, not after you develop a strong trusting relationship.

o **Do you like taking care of senior citizens?** Some doctors like to treat older people while others do not. Obviously you should find a doctor who enjoys serving you. In addition, the medical care given to older patients frequently differs from that given to someone who is younger, even though the disease or illness may be the same. It is in your interest that you choose a doctor who specializes in the care of senior citizens.

o **Do you take continuing education courses in geriatrics?** Medical Science is always avoiding information expanding at a fast pace. If your doctor is not keeping up with the changes in geriatric case management, he or she will become obsolete and you will be the one to suffer.

- Share your health history, including all illnesses in your immediate family.

- Tell your doctor about all the medication you are taking or have taken.

- Ask your doctor for recommendations for preventive care.

- Gat a copy of all test results for your personal file.

THE HOSPITAL

Sooner or later you or a loved one may have to spend some time in a hospital. There are hospitals that cater to the needs of the elderly. These are the ones you should visit. Assuming you have a choice, you should go to the hospital that pays optimum attention to your health and well-being.

Choosing Your Hospital

You can learn a lot about a hospital before you enter. One of the mot important criteria you should use to judge a hospital is the quality and delivery of its health services. This, in addition to its physical surrounding, should be of the highest standard. How do you find a hospital that fits this description? As it relates to the quality and delivery of health services, you should ask your doctor, friends, relatives or the hospital administration, the following questions to determine whether or not you want to visit that hospital.

- Ask your doctor why he or she is sending you to a particular hospital. Whether you are being treated by your primary health care physician or another doctor, it is his or her responsibility to recommend a hospital that is suited to your needs. Your choice is usually limited to one of the hospitals in which your doctor is permitted to practise, that is, where he is on staff. Your job, or that of the person who is assisting you, is to ensure that your doctor's recommendation is based on solid reasons, such as the quality of the nursing staff and other related services. The emphasis should be on your welfare and not just the convenience of the doctor. In addition, you should also find out whether the nurses are well trained and whether the hospital is well equipped to handle any complications you may experience.

- Ask your friends, relatives, doctors or medical professionals about their experiences with the particular hospital. Learning by "word of mouth" about the hospital may be as valuable as learning from those who are intimately involved with the facility. If you hear things that you are uncomfortable with, discuss it with your doctor.

- Ask the administration of several hospitals about the type and quality senior citizen services that they offer, and then compare.

Tips To Make Your Hospital Visit(s) Less Stressful

Going to the hospital can be a stressful event. The sights are not familiar, the language sounds strange, and the people are all new. No matter what the reason for the trip, whether it is an overnight visit for a few tests or a longer stay for a medical treatment or major surgery, nearly everyone is apprehensive about entering a hospital.

If you go to the hospital by choice or because of an emergency, the following information may make the trip less stressful. Also, relatives and friends of patients may find this information useful.

- *What to take with you to the hospital?*

  It is best to pack as little as possible and put your name on all personal items. Here are some items that you must pack:

  o Nightclothes, a bathrobe and sturdy slippers.

  o Comfortable clothes to wear home

  o Toiletries, including toothpaste, bath soap, tissue, etc.

  o A list of all the medicines you take, including prescription and non-prescription drugs.

  o Details of past illnesses, surgeries and any allergies.

  o Proof of any health insurance you may have.

o A list of names and telephone numbers (home and business) of family members to contact in case of an emergency.

o Money for newspapers, magazines or any other items you may wish to buy in the hospital gift shop.

- *What you should not take to the hospital?*

    o Cash

    o Jewelry (including wedding rings, earrings and watches)

    o Credit cards and cheque books. Ask a family member or friend to keep them. If you must bring valuables, ask if they can be kept in the hospital safety deposit box during your stay.

    o Electric razors, hair dryers and curling irons. They may not be compatible with the electrical wiring in the hospital grounded properly and could there be unsafe.

Hospital Procedures

- *Admission*

The first stop in the hospital is the Office of Admittance. Here, the patient or a family member signs forms which authorize the hospital staff to provide treatment and to release medical information to the insurance company. Those who do not have private health insurance can talk with an admissions counselor about other payment methods or source of financial aid.

- *Hospital Staff*

  After getting settled in your room, you should meet the members of your health care team.

  - o *Doctors*. They attend to each patient and are in charge of your overall care. It may be your regular doctor, one on the hospital staff, or a specialist. In teaching hospitals, you might be visited by the attending physician, along with medical students, interns and residents.

  - o *Nurses*. There are different types of nurses, such as registered nurses, nurse practitioners, licensed practical nurses, and nurses' aides. Nursing students also provide patient-care services.

  - o *Physical therapists*. They teach patients to build muscles and improve coordination. They may use exercise, heat, cold or water therapy to help patients whose ability to move is limited.

o *Occupational therapists*. They work with patients to restore, maintain or increase their ability, to perform daily tasks such as cooking, eating, bathing and dressing.

o Speech therapists work with patients who had a stroke or those recovering from throat surgery and neurosurgery.

o Respiratory therapists prevent and treat breathing problems.

o Technicians conduct a variety of laboratory tests, such as blood and urine tests and X-rays.

o Dieticians teach you how to plan a well-balanced diet.

o Pharmacists are educated in the chemical makeup and the correct use of drugs. They prepare the medicines you will take.

o Social workers offer support to patients and their families. They can provide details about how to obtain health care and social services after leaving the hospital, support groups and home-care services.

● *Patient-care Facilities*

Hospitals have many patient-care facilities. You

may be placed in a private room (one bed) or a semi-private (two bed) room. The intensive care unit (ICU) has special equipment and staff to care for very ill patients. In both the ICU, visiting hours are strictly limited and sometimes only family members are allowed to see patients. Surgery is done in the operating room (OR). After an operation, patients spend time in a recovery room.

In the emergency room (ER), trained staff treat life-threatening injuries or Illnesses. Patients who are badly injured or very ill are seen first. Because the ER is so busy, some patients may have to wait before they are seen by an emergency medical technician (paramedic), nurse or doctor.

- *Use of prosthetic appliances*

  A prosthetic appliance is used to care for patients with partial or total absence of a limb. In the event that you might use one, to maximize its use, ensure that you are instructed in proper usage. This will reduce the incidence of further injury.

- *Discharge*

  Before going home, you must get a discharge order from your doctor and a release form from the hospital's business office. Preparing for your discharge from the hospital can help you prepare for your health and home-care needs when you go home. This planning service is provided by a registered nurse, social worker or discharge planner. The discharge planner also knows about senior centres, nursing homes and other long-term care services.

- *Settling the cost of your healthcare*

  Before you leave the hospital, all outstanding bills for your medical care should be settled. These can be taken care of by your health insurance company, or by you. In the event that you are not able to do so, there are many non-profit organizations and other foundations whose function is to assist seniors (and others) who are victims of specific ailments. The Jamaica Heart Association and the Jamaica Cancer Society are two such groups. These organizations offer information and practical assistance to persons and are a great source of emotional and financial (for those in need) support.

Safety Tips

Because medical equipment may be unfamiliar and medications you take can make you feel tired or weak, it is necessary that you take a few extra safety precautions while you are in the hospital. These include:

- Use the call bell when you need help.

- Use the controls to lower the bed before getting in or out.

- Be careful not to trip over the many wires and tubes that may be around the bed.

- Try to keep the things you need within reach.

- Take only the medicine prescribed for you.

- If you brought your own medicine, tell your nurse or doctor, and take them only with your doctor's permission.

- Be careful when getting in and out of the bathtub or shower. Hold on to the grab bars for support. Ask for assistance.

- Use handrails on stairways and in hallways.

- Smoke only where allowed, and never smoke around oxygen.

Questions You Should Ask During Your Visit To The Hospital

During your hospital stay you may have many questions about your care. Always feel free to ask your doctor these questions. Your nurse or social worker may also be able to answer many of your questions or get the information you need. You may find it useful to write down your questions as you think of them. Examples are:

- What will this test tell you? Why is it needed?
- What treatment is needed, and how long will it last?
- What are the benefits and risks of the treatment?
- When can I go home?
- When I go home, will I have to change my regular activities?
- How often will I need checkups?
- Is any other follow-up care needed?
- Will I need physical therapy or occupational therapy?

THE PHARMACY

When you visit your doctor or the hospital, in most cases, you will get a prescription(s) for medication. The doctor sometimes will give you the medication that he has prescribed. However, in some instances, you will have to fill the prescription at a pharmacy -a place where drugs are sold or dispensed.

What You Should Do At The Pharmacy

- If convenient, use the same pharmacy for all your

prescriptions and ask the pharmacist (if possible) to keep a record of your medicines on the computer.

- Develop a personal relationship with the pharmacist.

- Ask the pharmacist to explain the instructions on your medication, for example, duration of treatment, dosage, side effects, etc.

Tips On Taking Your Medication

The medication that is prescribed will help to improve your health. You need to ask (your doctor or pharmacist) questions about the side effects, possible drug interactions and the precautionary measures that should be taken while you are on the medication. It is also important that you comply with the course treatment.

These are some tips to guide you:

- Ask for information concerning the side effects of a drug when you get a new prescription.

- Carry a card in your wallet or pocket book listing all the medications (both prescription and over-the-counter) that you are taking.

- Always check with your doctor before taking any new medication. If you have more than one doctor, each might be prescribing for you without the knowledge of other drugs that you are taking. It is therefore important that you inform each doctor about all the medication you are taking.

- If you drink alcohol, ask if it is safe to consume while you are taking a particular medication.

- If you are unsure of the names of, or the reasons why you are taking a particular drug, take them to your doctor so that he/she can explain.

- Make a chart, noting how often you are to take each medication, when (before or after meals), the name, and reason for taking it.

- Always check the label before you take any medication.

- Never take any medication in the dark. Ensure that you know what it is.

- Record the time you take your medication and when you should take it again, so you do not forget.

- Do not stop taking your medication because you start to feel better. Complete the total prescription, unless otherwise instructed by your doctor.

- Keep all medications in a dry and secure place.

- Throw out all old medication, as they deteriorate with age, rendering them ineffective.

Senior Citizens at Worship, Work & Play

At Worship

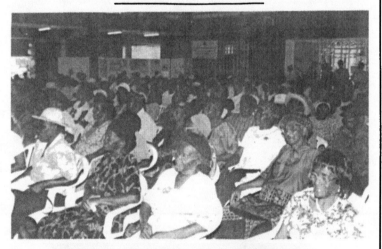

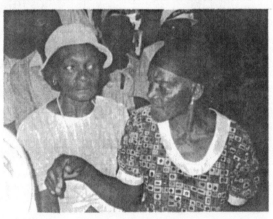

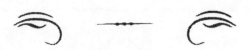

WHERE TO GET HELP

There are a number of places in Jamaica where senior citizens can go to get assistance, ranging from payment for medication to transportation.

NATIONAL COUNCIL FOR SENIOR CITIZEN (NCSC)

Location: 11 West Kings House Road, Kingston 10
Telephone: (876) 926-2374/5, 906-9277/8

The NCSC and the Ministry of Health (Jamaica), have the following services to which senior citizens can go to for assistance.

Drugs For The Elderly Programme

- This programme benefits people 60 years and older, and who are in need of assistance to pay for their medication.

At Work

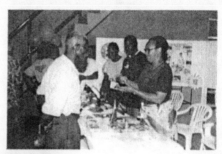

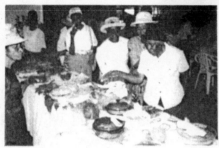

At Play

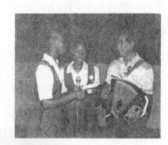

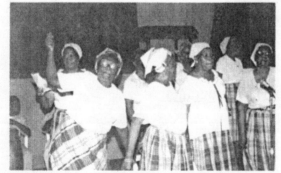

- If you meet these requirements, visit the Ministry of Health or the health centre nearest to you, and fill out an application.

- Take along some form of identification to verify your age. If you do not have any form of identification, ask a Justice of the Peace, your pastor or doctor to write a letter, verifying your age. Take this letter along with you when you go to fill out the application.

- When the process is completed (on same day if you go to the Ministry of Health or up to 7 days if you go to your local health center), you will receive a blue card, which you should take with you when you visit the pharmacy.

- The card is effective for only three years, after which it should be renewed.

- Only drugs on the approved list will be covered under the programme. If you buy 1 to 2 drugs, you pay J$25.00; 3 to 4, you pay J$50.00; and 5 to 6 you pay J$75.00.

Transportation Assistance Programme

This service is available for senior citizens, 60 years and older. You get a bus pass that you present to the conductor upon entering the bus. It entitles you to pay only J$10.00.

NATIONAL INSURANCE SCHEME (NIS)

Location: 18 Ripon Road
                Kingston 5
                Telephone: (876) 929-7119, 929-7122

Pension

You are eligible to receive pension from the NIS if you had contributed to it while you were working. Upon retirement, age 65 years for men and 60 years for women, you can apply for benefits.

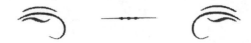

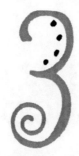

3

TO STAY OR GO?

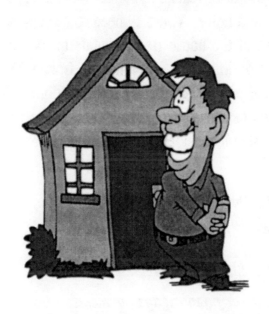

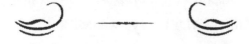

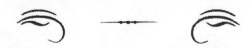

TYPES OF LIVING ARRANGEMENTS

You do not have to change your living arrangements because you have reached your retirement age and/or your kids have left home. You may need some support and assistance around the house if you decide to live alone. There are many options that are available from which you can choose (see page 30 for further information). However, if you decide to stay in your own home, buy a new home or rent, you should consider the following factors.

STAYING IN YOUR OWN HOME
Sometimes no move is the best move!

Advantages Of Staying In Your Own Home

- *Little or no mortgage payments.*

    This means you will have more money to do or buy the things you always wanted to.

- *Maintaining your roots.*

  Psychologists agree that most people live a better quality of life if they feel stable and secure in their surroundings. So staying in an environment where you know the neighbours or have family may greatly add to your well-being. Knowing the 'lay of the land,' or your environment also builds confidence and makes chores around the house easier. Growing older should mean happy memories and memories are perhaps best enjoyed in the place they were created.

- *It eliminates the stress of moving.*

  Change causes stress for everyone, particularly older persons. It takes time and energy, and can be expensive. The experience may prove to be more harmful than beneficial.

- *Income opportunities.*

  You can always earn extra money (and companion-ship) by renting a room to someone with whom you feel safe and are compatible.

- *Freedom.*

  You are free to do anything you want and to make your own decisions when you are in your own home.

- *Tax benefits.*

When you make your house payment, most of the interest is to mortgage lender. The good news is that this interest, as well as the money paid on property tax is tax deductible. This translates into a tax break.

- *Increased property value.*

Property values tend to rise. These 'paper profits' can easily be converted into cash.

- *Stability.*

Buying a home means buying into a neighbourhood that will most likely remain relatively stable for an extended period of time. You can buy a mortgage or trust deed payment that will either never change (such as a fixed rate loan), or you get a variable rate loan that ideally will rise or fall slowly over the years. You should buy in a location in which all the necessary amenities are in place and are unlikely to change during the time you are living there.

- *Intangibles.*

Finally, there is something special about saying "this is my home" and owning your own space. Nobody can take that away from you.

BUYING A NEW HOME

The home that was appropriate when your family lived

with you may be too large or too far from the hospital, doctor, or other facilities that become more important as you grow older. You may be having trouble maintaining your home or the community has changed. Perhaps your children live in a different parish or country and you want to be closer to them. Whatever the reason for moving, you should ask yourself some questions before deciding to buy a new house or relocating.

Questions You Should Ask Yourself

The following are some questions you should ask yourself if you are going to buy a new home:

- *Can I handle the responsibilities that come with buying a new home?*

    Owning a house is a big responsibility. It requires a lot of your time and attention and it could impinge on your leisure time. For example, you may have to do chores around the house when you could be playing a game of tennis. You may be reluctant to travel for fear of leaving the house unattended for long periods. Also the financial cost of maintaining a home after retirement may be too great a burden.

- *Can I afford to buy?*

    There is more to buying a house than paying the price monthly loan payment you may have to make. For example there is the down payment and closing costs, maintenance, house repairs and unexpected costs, such as special assessment or hurricane damage, plus the expense of furnishing a new home. In fact, the financial burden may be heavier than you first expected.

- *Will I feel secure in my own home?*

When you own a home, you are more susceptible to vandalism and theft, than your counterparts who may live in apartments where security services are provided.

RENTING

For those who want to avoid the expense and responsibility of home ownership, renting can be an option. There are no lawns to mow or toilets to repair, as these are the responsibilities of the landlord. There is usually less space in an apartment than a house, so housework takes less time. You simply pay the rent and maintain the place and the landlord is legally bound to do the rest.

Questions You Should Ask Yourself

If you intend to rent an apartment, consider the following before you do so:

- *How much will you be paying each month for rent and how often will the amount increase?*

Be sure you understand the terms of your lease before you sign, so that you are not surprised by any unexpected rent increases. You should also find out your legal rights and obligations, so you can protect yourself in the event your landlord conveniently forgets the rules.

- *Do you want to lease or rent?*

A lease is a contract between you and the owner, which gives you the right to live on the premises for a fixed period of time at a fixed rental price. A lease protects you from rent increases during the term of agreement and from eviction, provided you abide by the terms of the contract.

There are certain terms and conditions in the lease agreement that you must understand before it is signed. For example, if you want to move before the lease expires, the landlord can sue you for rent lost due to breach of the terms of the lease agreement. There will also be a "renewal clause" in your lease contract, which allows you to stay under the terms of the lease. It is important to note that in most cases when a lease contract is renewed, there is often an increase in the rental amount, which is usually based on a financial guideline that is stated in the lease itself. As a result, if you intend to renew the contract, ensure that you understand it and the legal consequences of signing. It is usually a good idea to get a lawyer to review the terms of the proposed lease and explain it to you before you sign it.

- *Will the landlord maintain the property?*

Inspect the apartment you are renting to ensure that everything, including light switches, fixtures in the bathroom and kitchen are in proper working condition. In the event that they are not, be sure to write in the rental agreement that the landlord is obligated to repair them before you move in.

- *Does the owner of the property live on the premises?*

A "live-in" manager can respond to your needs faster than one who only visits when the rent is due. You should always get the name and address of the actual owner so that you have someone to call if you are unhappy with the way your apartment is being managed, or if there are any other problems.

BOARD AND CARE

For seniors who may not like or cannot afford the choices listed above, board and care is another option. It is for those seniors who need assistance on a daily basis, but do not want to stay in a nursing home. This type of residence is similar to shared housing except you are provided with meals and assistance with grooming.

TYPES OF SERVICES
THAT ARE AVAILABLE TO ASSIST CAREGIVERS

Most caregivers prefer to offer their services in the home of the person that they are caring for. If the caregiver is a spouse, an effort should be made to keep the loved one at home in familiar environs for as long as possible. If the caregiver is an offspring, he or she may decide to take the parent to his/her home. Either way, caregivers should be aware of the types of services that are available to assist them. This will reduce their level of stress and frustration.

HOSPICE CARE

If you are caring for a senior with a terminal illness, you can use the services of a hospice to assist you and your loved one during this time. The services are designed to make your life as a caregiver easier. For additional information, see section entitled, *'When your spouse is terminally ill.'*

HOME HEALTH CARE

This may become necessary for senior citizens who need ongoing medical care. If you are going to keep a loved one at home, you must learn to give medical care yourself (where appropriate) or use in-home health care services, or both. It could be a registered nurse who makes house calls and performs services that a nurse in a hospital would perform, such as changing dressings, giving injections or performing catheter care; or you or your family learning to administer oxygen or insulin.

What To Look For When Choosing In-home Healthcare Companies

- *A company your doctor trusts.*

- *A company that provides training for its staff in new techniques.* New medical techniques and equipment are always evolving and doctors are not the only ones who have to keep abreast of these new developments. You need a company that trains its professionals in the latest techniques and on the latest equipment.

- *A company that is licensed.*

  While this may not be a guarantee of quality, it is better than nothing.

For more information on these services, contact your local health care agencies, public health departments, churches, day care centres, or area agencies on ageing.

How To Make Your Home More Comfortable For you And Your Loved One(s)

The following are some tips to help you to make your home more comfortable for you and your loved one(s).

- If possible, provide the older person with his or her own room or space where they can spend time in private. Ideally, the room should be on the first floor to avoid the necessity of climbing stairs.

- Encourage your loved one to participate in home activities. For example, doing chores and other activities that are within their capabilities.

- Ensure that your loved one has a social life as his/her health permits. Senior-citizen centres in your area should be consulted to see what programmes are available.

- Install safety fixtures such as handrails next to the toilet and shower. A bench should also be placed in the bathtub for easy and safe access.

- Install wrist straps on the walker or cane to reduce the chances of a fall.

- Remove all shag carpets and throw rugs to prevent slipping or falling.

- If the person has physical challenges, consider about installing side rails on the sides of the bed. This will help prevent him or her from falling out of bed and makes getting out of bed easier.

NURSING HOME CARE

There may come a time when, for whatever reasons, an older person simply must be placed in a long-term nursing care facility, also known as a nursing home. This decision is never an easy one. Some nursing homes have earned the reputation of being places where seniors are warehoused, rather than provided with quality custodial care. However, there are many nursing homes that do provide excellent care.

The problem, of course, is to find them. After all, most of us do not spend our spare time thinking about the advantages/disadvantages of nursing home care. If or when we do, it is usually when we are in a crisis, and this is usually not the best time to make such an important decision.

Choosing A Nursing Home

The following are some important things to consider:

- *Ensure that you understand what you are paying for.*

  Nursing homes provide four basic services:

o Medical care is usually provided by the patient's doctor, who admits him or her to the nursing home and who remains personally responsible for the patient's continuing treatment.

o Nursing care by Registered Nurses (RNs), who administer medicine, injections, catheterizations, among others, as ordered by a doctor.

o Personal care, such as assistance in walking, bathing, eating, dressing and the preparation of special diets as ordered by a physician.

o Residential services including general supervision and protection, room and board, and a program of social and recreational activities.

The level and quality of service will vary from nursing home to nursing home. You want a home that provides the best mix of services to meet your loved one's needs, both at the time of admission and if his or her condition worsens.

● *Plan Ahead.*

If you are the care-giver for a senior citizen, it is important that you find out about the nursing homes within or near your community, before you actually need one, or in the event that you might need one. In doing so, you will have enough time to find a home which is best suited to the specific needs of your loved one.

- *Know the Rights of Nursing Home Patients.*

  When looking into nursing home facilities, make sure the administrators take the following patients' rights seriously:

  o The rights to safe and considerate cares.

  o An environment which is clean and in good hygienic condition.

  o A diet consisting of a variety of good quality foods as prescribed by the patient's physician.

  o The presence of organized social and physical activities.

  o The right to privacy when visited by a spouse and the right to share a room if both spouses are residents of the facility.

  o Liberal visiting hours on a daily basis.

  o An environment in which grievances may be presented without fear of reprisals.

  o Dignity and respect in personal care.

  o An environment that allows for freedom of religious expression and worship.

o An opportunity for the patients to purchase drugs and medical supplies from a pharmacy or other source of their choice.

- *Check the Cost.*

Nursing homes offer different prices for their services. It is therefore important that you choose the one that is affordable, as it is no secret that many nursing home patients have literally become bankrupt while paying for their care. This fact of life compels the caregiver to look into payment options, such as, by the family, legal/financial planning or alternate sources of payment, such as insurance.

- *Check the Location.*

One of the best ways to ensure that your loved one receives the best care is to visit the location on a regular basis. In order to do this, you should find a good nursing home that is relatively close to you.

- *Check the Facilities*

When you are choosing a nursing home, you should compare and contrast facilities just as you would when choosing any product or service. Look carefully for the following:

o *Licensing.* Ensure that the nursing home has all the necessary legal licences and whether the administrator's licence is up to date. Also check if the most current license report is posted in a prominent location, as it will outline problems that were found in the last inspection, and if there were, if these were corrected.

o *Atmosphere and treatment of residents.* Look at the general atmosphere of the nursing home and note if it is pleasant and cheerful. Do the staff seem enthusiastic and genuinely interested in their patients? Are the residents properly cared for and are they allowed basic freedoms, such as decorating their rooms, or have privacy during family visits? Ask around and see whether other visitors and volunteers speak favourably about the home.

o *General physical considerations.* The nursing home should be clean and orderly and relatively free from unpleasant odours. The rooms should be well ventilated and kept at a comfortable temperature.

o *Safety procedures.* Check to see if wheelchair ramps are provided where necessary and whether the hallways and bathrooms are equipped with grab bars and hand-rails. Also check to see if bathtubs and showers have non-slip surfaces and note if the nursing home is generally free of obvious hazards such as obstacles or unsteady furniture. Make a note of how well prepared the home seems at handling unexpected disasters such as fires. Are there smoke detectors and portable fire extinguishers? Are exits clearly marked, are the doors free from obstacles and are able to be unlocked from the inside? Are emergency evacuation plans posted in conspicuous locations?

o *Medical and dental services.* Are arrangements made with outside dental services to provide patients with dental care when necessary? How does the home handle a medical emergency? Ask if there is a physician available at all times (either on staff or on call) and whether they have arrangements with a nearby hospital for quick transfer of nursing home patients. Is emergency transportation readily available?

o *Pharmaceutical services.* Does a licensed pharmacist supervise pharmaceutical supplies? Is a pharmacist employed to maintain and monitor a record of each patient's drug therapy? Is a room set aside for storing and preparing drugs? Does the facility encourage purchase of drugs from the supplier of your choice?

o *Nursing services.* Check to see that an RN is on duty during the day, seven days a week. Find out if at least one RN is on duty at nights. Are nurse or emergency call buttons located at each patient's bed and in toilet and bathing facilities?

o *Food preparation and delivery.* Make sure that the kitchen is clean and reasonably tidy and that waste is properly disposed of. Check to see if the dining room is attractive and comfortable. Ask to see the meal schedule and check to see that at least three meals are provided each day. Find out if the meal being served matches the posted menu. Also note if meals are served at normal hours, with plenty of time for leisurely eating. Are patients given enough food? Are nutritious snacks available? Are special meals prepared for residents on a restricted diet? Ensure that assistance is available for those who need assistance with eating.

o *Social services and patient activities.* Find out if the home has a varied programme of recreational, cultural and intellectually stimulating activities for patients and ask if there is an activities director on staff. Are there special activities for those confined to their rooms? Are there social services to aid patients and their families?

o *Patient's rooms.* Does each room have a window and open into a hallway? Does each patient have a reading light, a comfortable chair and drawers for personal belongings? Is there fresh drinking water within reach? Is there a curtain or screen available to provide privacy for each bed whenever necessary? Do bathing facilities and toilets have adequate privacy?

o *Other areas in the nursing home.* Check to see if there is a lounge area where patients can chat, read, play games, watch television or just relax outside of their rooms. Is there an outdoor area where patients can get fresh air and sunshine? Find out if there is a public telephone available for patients' use.

o *Financial and related matters.* Compare the estimated monthly costs, including extra charges, with the cost of other homes. Check if there is a refund policy for monies paid in advance and the facility was not used. Ensure that these matters are clearly set out in the written contract.

Know what to do if there is a problem.

No one wants to be involved in a dispute. But imagine if you were ill, confined to a nursing home and you were involved in a dispute with those responsible for your care. Imagine the fear you would have of confronting those responsible for your comfort and health and, perhaps, even your life. Under these circumstances, the patient should not be the one that deals with the situation. A member of the family or a friend of the family should be appointed to communicate with the patient and intercede on his or her behalf when necessary. If a family member refuses to undertake the responsibility, hire a private geriatric care manager to do the investigation on your behalf.

Here are some tips to help you in the event you become unhappy with the care of your loved one:

o *Talk privately to the person involved in the problem.* Before calling in the "big guns", such as the director of nursing, have a private chat with the person with whom your loved one has a dispute. You might be surprised that there are two sides to the controversy and how receptive he or she can be in trying to alleviate the problem.

o *Take the matter to the top.* If talking with the person does not help, speak with the next person in command, such as the director of nursing of the facility or the administrator or both. Remember, you are paying for a service of which the administrator is aware. He/she is obligated to positively respond to the problems you bring to his/her attention.

o *Report the home to the authorities.* If the problem is very serious, such as abuse, patient neglect or unsanitary facilities, report the home to the health department and licensing authorities.

o *Avoid problems in the first place.* The best way to solve problems is to identify potentially troublesome areas and deal with them before they become problems. This is best done by visiting often and ensuring that your loved one is receiving quality care. (For example, the existence of bedsores might indicate that a bedridden patient is not being turned often enough). It is also a very good idea to humanize the patient in the staffs mind. For instance, you could put a picture of the patient, taken in better times, and hang it up on his or her door with a list of accomplishments reminding everyone that this enfeebled and dependent person was once a vital and productive member of society and, as such, deserves respect and gentle care.

CARING FOR PATIENTS WITH ALZHEIMER'S DISEASE

Alzheimer's disease deserves special mention because of its prevalence and the quality of care that its victims require. This incurable disease destroys the brain's memory and the body's ability to maintain its own existence. As the disease advances, the victim's mental and physical state deteriorates. The caregiver therefore experiences more challenges to care for such individual.

If you are a caregiver for a patient with Alzheimer's disease, it is important that you get legal and financial advice. If they live long enough, victims of Alzheimer's disease will eventually become incapacitated by the disease. The cost of maintaining a decent level of care for victims, whether at home or in a nursing facility is expensive. Lawyers who specialize in laws that concern senior citizens and financial planners can help manage the family assets. You may also want to get some advice on estate planning in the event that something unfortunate should happen to your patient.

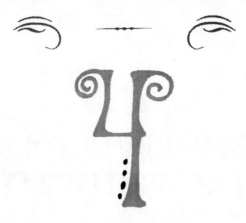

Dealing with the **not so** pleasant aspects of the **GOLDEN YEARS**

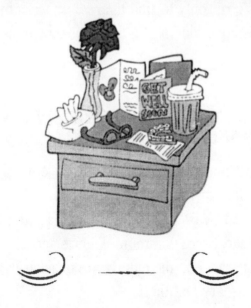

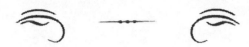

SAFEGUARDING YOUSELF AGAINST VICTIMIZATION

There should be a reward given to everyone who lives a long life and reaches 'seniordom'. After all, longevity does not happen by accident. It takes effort, and a little bit of luck, to overcome the wars, diseases, and accidents, that face us in our daily lives. There are those among us who achieve this goal, only to find themselves beset by fears, of which becoming a victim of a crime or scheme is at the top of the list.

COMMON SHEMES AND ACTS OF CRIMES THAT YOU SHOULD BE AWARE OF

There are many dishonest people in our midst. They particularly like to prey on the elderly, as they are more vulnerable and least likely to report a crime, usually because of fear. Some common schemes and acts of crimes that are perpetrated on the elderly are quackery, scams and cons, and burglary and theft.

<u>Quackery</u>

This is the promotion of a medical remedy that has not been proven to work. In legal terms, it is fraud. The person, who perpetrates this form of fraud, often promises miracle cures and overnight results, even though they do not exist. It is a dishonest activity, because it preys on people's fears. At best, quackery takes your money; at worst, it takes your life.

Senior citizens are usually susceptible to this practice, because they are the most vulnerable members of society. It is therefore important that you protect yourself from individuals who practise this fraudulent activity.

The following are some of the more common conditions that people involved in this type of fraud claim to have cures for:

- *Arthritis*

  Life can be difficult to those afflicted with arthritis. Its symptoms may be relieved, it may even go into periods of remission, but the unfortunate truth is that arthritis is incurable. Anyone promising a cure is a quack. As for the treatment of pain and inflammation, there are legitimate and illegitimate methods. Before you accept any treatment, ensure that a reputable doctor or health organization has approved it.

- *Cancer*

  Victims and the family members of victims of cancer are prime targets for quackery. Quacks thrive on the misfortune of others, and there is none more serious than a family member being stricken with cancer. People become so desperate they will believe anything.

  The quack often hypes "miracle machines" to cure cancer. Others fan the flames of paranoia and accuse the medical community of suppressing the cure. They often urge the victims to leave the country and attend their clinics. Be aware of any cancer treatment that a reputable doctor refuses to administer to his or her patient.

- *Weight Loss*

  We would all like to be able to eat everything and still lose weight or lose weight while we sleep. However, we can lose weight only if we reduce our calorie intake, exercise regularly or both. Any "breakthrough" drug, weight loss tonic or device that claims otherwise, should be avoided.

- *Impotence*

  Sexual dysfunction is a condition that everyone is uncomfortable with. It can be caused by physical or psychological factors, but it can be cured. However, it is not cured by powders, drugs or a hormone replacement therapy. If you are impotent, consult your doctor. If the problem is not of a physical nature, seek treatment from a licensed therapist, who is trained to deal with sexual dysfunction.

There is probably a fraudulent scheme for every ailment known to man, from hair loss to the common cold. The following are some of the more common promotional devices used by quacks to fool their victims:

- Mail order offers with a money back guarantee. Very often your letter requesting a refund will be returned with "return to sender".

- Testimonials from "satisfied users": If they sound too good to be true, they usually are.

- Promises of "quick and painless cures": Being cheated out of your money may be quick, but never painless.

- Advertisements of "scientific breakthroughs" and "miracle cures" or "secret ancient formulas." Mail order products or products advertised in the newspaper with these descriptions are worth less than the paper on which they are printed.

You should be very aware, especially when it comes to your health. If you are interested in any health care product, call your primary care physician and ask for his or her advice. Another person to consult is your pharmacist. If he or she cannot confirm the merits of the treatment, it is probably a scam.

Scams And Con Games

Older people are the prime targets for scam artistes, because of the following reasons:

- Older people find it harder to identify the perpetrator of the crime.

- Older people do not react as quickly to impropriety.

- Older people tend to stay in the con longer because they tend to be more trusting, especially if the person appears to be sincere.

- Older people are generally more susceptible to pressure.

- Older people are more reluctant to say no.

- Once conned, older people are reluctant to come forward to report the crime. In fact, many keep the con a secret for fear that they will be thought senile or incapable of taking care of themselves.

The word *'artiste'* is very appropriate, as these men and women are artistes, dramatic actors who are very skilled professionals. Their main purpose is to get you to trust or feel sorry for them, or to convince you to give them your money, credit card number or other form of valuable personal belongings. It is important to note that con artists are not easily recognizable, as they come in many disguises.

Burglary And Theft

Perhaps one of the greatest fears that an older person faces is, that of becoming the victim of a violent crime or theft. Older people are frequently the targets of criminals and thieves, as they are less likely to defend themselves against an attack. However, this does not mean that you should not take the necessary precautions to protect yourself. If you do so, the risks of becoming a crime statistic are greatly reduced.

- *Burglary*

    Burglary is defined as the crime of breaking into and entering a building with the intention of stealing. Typically, the burglar enters the victim's home and steals property to be later sold for cash. However, most burglaries can be prevented. The best defence is good offence. Here are some tips for defending your home against burglars:

    o   Always lock your doors and windows whenever you leave home, even if you will be away for a short period of time. It takes a short period of time for a thief to invade your space.

o Doors on the outside should have a deadbolt lock that extends into the doorframe. Simple push-button locks are almost useless.

o Sliding doors and windows should have special locks installed. You can drill a hole through the door and metal frame and put in a thick screw.

o Ensure that gates and grilles are locked.

o If you are leaving your home, use timers on the lights, radio and television set to go on and off at varied intervals. This gives the impression that someone is home. If these are not available, keep your radio on.

o If you will be away on a long trip, stop the delivery of mail and newspaper until you return. Newspapers and mail that are not picked up are like gold-plated invitations to anyone who wish to commit a crime.

o Install a wide-angle lens viewer in the front door. Never open the door unless you know who is there.

o Personalize your valuables by marking them with your driver's licence number or date of birth. Marked items have no value on the black market and may be left behind. Take pictures of all valuables you keep at home for insurance purposes. If you have access to a safety deposit box, use it to store valuables and other important documents.

o Whenever you move to a new house, change the locks.

o Ensure your property is well lit during the night.

o Consider installing an alarm or a security device.

o If you come home and your door is open or there are other indications of forcible entry, do not go into the house! Most burglars do not want a confrontation, but may turn violent when caught. Remember, life is more valuable than your property.

Please note: If your home is burglarized, call the police. Your may never get back the stolen items, but unless you report the crime, your insurance company will not pay for your losses. In addition, the police have a chance of catching the perpetrator if they are made aware of the crime.

Theft or robbery

Theft is the unlawful act of taking another person's property. Robbery is an act or an instance of unlawfully taking the property of another by the use of violence or intimidation. Both robbers and thieves consider senior citizens easy preys.

Here are some tips to protect you from becoming a victim of thieves and robbers:

o If you carry a purse, hold it close to your body. Do not dangle it. To do so is to literally give someone an invitation to snatch it.

o Never carry your wallet in your back pocket, put it in an inside jacket pocket or front pocket.

o Let someone know where you are going and when you are expected to return.

o Do not travel dark or deserted routes alone, and if it cannot be avoided, travel in large numbers, as there is safety in numbers.

o Have your key in hand as you approach your car or home.

o Do not carry many packages that obstruct your view and prevent you from reacting to danger.

o Carry a whistle with you wherever you go so

that you can attract attention if you are being robbed.

o Use traveller's cheques instead of cash to minimize your loss, since you can be compensated for lost or stolen traveler's cheques. You should also use credit cards and bank cards whenever possible.

o When you drive, keep your windows up and your doors locked. Park in well-lit areas and be wary of strangers asking for help. Instead, offer to call the police or a tow truck when you get home.

o If a friend or a taxi takes you home, ask them to wait until you are safely inside before they leave.

o When walking, act calm and confident. Trust your gut feelings. If your internal danger alarm begins to sound, be extra careful.

o If you are attacked, do not resist if the assailant is only after your purse. If you resist, chances are you will be hurt. If the attack is more personal, defend yourself in any way you can. Check with a crime prevention programme, such as a neighbourhood watch programme in your area for more details and information about how to keep yourself safe.

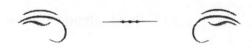

PUTTING YOUR AFFAIRS IN ORDER

Death is inevitable. The least we can do is prepare for it, by ensuring that our affairs are in order and that our family members and friends know what to do when it happens.

THE PROBATE SYSTEM

While we are alive, we accumulate money, property and other material possessions that make up our estate. When we die, these are left behind. Your estate is then probated. A probate is a legal action that takes place in Probate Court. The purpose is to distribute your property among the living, (either to the persons directed by you in a legal document called a will, or by the law to your nearest relatives). However, before it is distributed, your estate will be valued, your debts paid, estate taxes levied and fees subtracted from the estate to pay for lawyers and executors who are employed to carry out your wishes.

These fees and taxes can account for a large part of the estate; approximately 20-25% of the net market value of the estate. As a result, most people prefer to have their estate distributed as they have specified in their will to minimize estate taxes. Here is a general overview of the different ways in which this can be done.

Wills

Where there's a will and a lawyer, there is usually a way!

There are different types of wills, from the simple to the complicated. The purpose of a will is to direct the court to dispose of your property and personal possessions as stated in the document. A will can also name the person or persons you want to be the guardians of your children should you die before they are adults. Moreover, the provisions of a will can be used to reduce probate expenses on your estate. It can also be used to disinherit anyone who would otherwise be entitled to a share of your property.

The following are some general principles that need to be discussed when you are preparing a will.

● *Validity of handwritten will.*

A handwritten will, also known as a holographic will, is valid in most cases. Most people try to avoid the cost of a lawyer by writing their wills without legal consultation. However, it is valid only if it is entirely handwritten, dated and signed by the person making the will. The terms and conditions of the document must be clear, or it may be ruled invalid by the court. A holographic will does not have to be witnessed, but is more enforceable if it is.

Handwritten wills can be problematic in some instances. The following are some problems that are associated with handwritten wills.

o   Failure to use the proper legal language, which can result in all or part of the document deemed invalid by the court. This, in most cases, translates into additional money charged to your estate when it is probated, as a lawyer now has to be retained to interpret the document.

o   If there are any obliterations, interlineations or markings on a will, such as a line drawn through a word, sentence, or phrase, which are not initialed by the testator and the attesting witnesses to the will, a court may rule that the amendments to the will is invalid.

o   Disappointed heirs are more likely to challenge a handwritten will than a will prepared by lawyers, as the latter tends to be more binding.

- *Formal wills -from the simple to the complex.*

  These range from simple to complex. A formal will can be defined as one that is prepared by a lawyer, typed, dated, signed and witnessed, as required by the law. Formal wills can be simple, such as stating that you leave the entire estate to your spouse, or whomever you choose, and upon his or her death, to your children. Or they can be very complex with many built in contingencies and/or the creation of multiple trusts which can last for decades. A simple will is relatively inexpensive to prepare, while a very complicated document can be very expensive.

- *A will allows you to name the person you trust the most to manage your estate during probate.*

  When the estate is in probate court, someone has to be appointed by the court to manage the estate, pay the outstanding bills and take the necessary action to enforce the terms and conditions of the will. The person or financial institution, which is appointed, is called the executor, if named in the will, and an administrator if appointed by the court when a will is not made. This is a position of responsibility, as evidenced by the fact that many estates have deteriorated because of poor management.

- *Only one will is valid.*

  You can draft as many wills in your lifetime as you

wish, but only the last one is valid (assuming that it has been properly prepared and witnessed). The very act of writing a new will voids all previously drafted wills.

- *Wills can be revoked at any time*

   Assuming you are of sound mind and that no legal obstacles exist that could prevent you from revoking or invalidating your will (such as mental incompetence), you may do so at any time, by destroying, defacing it, or simply writing a new one.

- *A properly prepared will is very difficult to challenge.*

   If you believe that the provisions of your will are likely to create problems and the possibility of a lawsuit to invalidate its terms (for example, if you intend to disinherit a child or other close relative), be sure that a lawyer prepares your will. He or she should be able to draft a will that is legally binding. Wills are judged on the basis of their language. A poorly drafted will may have lots of loopholes, thereby increasing the likelihood of a challenge in court.

- *Wills can be modified.*

   You can write a new will at any time. However, if the changes you wish to make are relatively minor, you may not have to go to the expense of drafting an entirely new document. Instead, you can add a codicil that makes the changes you want, while the rest of the document remains unchanged.

- *Wills revoked by marriage*

A marriage will automatically revoke an existing will, so as soon as this occurs the couple should remake their wills.

Estate Planning

One of the problems with a will is that in order for it to be enforced, it usually has to be probated and this can be very expensive. However, one of the things you can do before you die is to arrange it so that the expense of probate or death taxes can be minimized. This is sometimes easier said than done, but it can be achieved, by doing what is referred to as "estate planning." The following are some options:

- *The living trust.*

The living trust eliminates the process of probate and saves the estate thousands of dollars in attorney's fees and probate costs. It can be very complicated, and most lawyers do not understand how it works.

However, simply put, the living trust has a "trustor," which is the person setting up the trust (you), who transfers all of his or her property into a legal entity known as a trust. A person known as a "trustee", again you, controls the property of the trust. In this case, legally, you no longer own the property (the trust does), but you do control it as long as you have made yourself the trustee. If you appoint someone else as the trustee, that person controls the property.

The trust is established to benefit the persons who are specifically named by you. These persons are called "beneficiaries." You can be the beneficiary or you can name others, called "alternate beneficiaries," to assume responsibility for the trust when you die. This means that during your lifetime, all your possessions will go to the trust. It also means that those persons, whom you have named as alternate beneficiaries, will inherit the property, without it being subjected to the process of probate. The reason why this is legal is that technically you did not own the property; therefore it cannot be probated upon your death.

Living trusts, however, are not perfect. Estate taxes can be applied and creditors can put a lien on the property to force the payment of debts. However, these conditions do not apply if the estate is in probate, as there is a relatively short period of time for creditors to state their claim. Living trusts, especially when compared to wills, can be expensive, as the former have to be prepared by a lawyer. But for many, the living trust is the most effective method of keeping your estate intact. You are also better able to maintain complete control over your property during your lifetime.

It is imperative that you retain the services of a lawyer to prepare a will to go with the trust. This will ensure that properties that are not named in the trust are taken care of.

- *Testamentary trust*

  A testamentary trust is one that is created in your will and comes into effect upon your death. The principal purpose of a testamentary trust is to minimize estate taxes and to control the manner in which your money is spent.

  A testamentary trust can also be used to protect the inheritors from themselves, by a stipulation that he or she receives a specific sum of money over a period of time.

  There are many other examples of testamentary trusts, so you should ask your lawyer for more information. In addition, unlike living trusts, testamentary trusts have to be probated. However, if you have a large estate, you can set up a testamentary trust, as this will protect you from high taxation.

- *Joint tenancy*

  Many people try to avoid the process of probate by placing their property, especially real estate, in joint tenancy. When one tenant dies, the surviving tenant automatically becomes the owner of the property. This is referred to as "the right of survivorship." This effectively eliminates the process of probate, since legally the deceased no longer has an ownership interest in the property.

  Whereas joint tenancy has its advantages, there are some disadvantages that you should be aware of.

  o You cease to have exclusive control over the property when another person's name is added as joint tenant. He or she automatically becomes an equal owner. This means that you would have to get the joint tenant's permission to sell the property. If he or she refuses, the matter would have to be taken to the court to force a sale. After which, you would receive your half of the funds when the attorney's fees and other costs have been subtracted.

o   When someone becomes a co-owner of your property, he or she could force you to sell.

o   If one of the joint tenants is in debt, creditors may subject his or her share of the property to liens.

o   You will have to pay estate taxes.

o   If you are interested in using joint tenancy, retain the services of a lawyer to draft a contract, stipulating the terms and conditions of the joint tenancy. In doing so, you can protect yourself from some of the problems associated with this method.

- *Gift giving*

One very effective way of reducing the cost of probate and estate taxes is to give the property as a gift to those whom you would have left to when you die. The taxes would be lower on your estate because it was given as a gift.

If you are interested in this method, you should be aware of the following:

o   If you give more than a certain amount per year in cash or property to anyone, a charitable or non-charitable organization, it will be subject to a gift tax. However, if you want to reduce the level of taxation, you should give the property or monies to as much people or organization as is legally possible.

o Certain gifts given within three years of death may still be subjected to estate taxes. The most common example of this is life insurance policies. There are also other types of gifts. Such as, forgiveness of a debt or the institution of an irrevocable trust (one which cannot be taken back). Giving someone the permission to withdraw money you have deposited in a joint bank account is also considered a gift.

o When a gift has been legally "given", you cannot take it back. A gift is considered given if a mentally competent person voluntarily delivers the gift to the person. Once the person accepts it, the transaction is complete, and you cannot change your mind or legally force a return of the gift.

o Giving gifts to children, who are considered minors, can be a complicated process, as the law stipulates that property owned by minors must be supervised by an adult. This usually involves the appointment of a custodian, such as a relative or a financial institution, who will manage the property on behalf of the minor until he or she reaches the legal age. Be sure to consult a lawyer before you give a substantial gift to a minor.

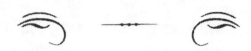

PREPARING FOR THE WORST

At one time or another, many older people are temporarily or permanently afflicted by diseases or disabilities, which may prevent them from making important decisions concerning their health and well-being. If the necessary arrangements are not made, such events can have far-reaching implications. Oftentimes, a vacuum is created where no one is in charge of the person's affairs. This can lead to a 'mad scramble' to "put things in order", which can cause conflict in the family.

If you are prepared for these eventualities, you can eliminate the conflict that might ensue. In addition, even if you are incapacitated, you will still have some amount of control over the decisions to be made.

CHOOSING TO LIVE OR TO DIE

While most of us fear death, it almost does not compare

to the helplessness we feel if we are kept alive by extraordinary measures. How can we ensure that this does not happen? Should we rely on our loved ones to inform the doctor to "pull the plug?" And if they do, are we not inadvertently inflicting a lifetime of guilt, as they will no doubt question their decision.

Fortunately, you can make that decision by:

- *Informed consent*

  Every patient who is legally competent to make a decision has the absolute right to decide the type of medical treatment he or she will or will not pursue. Under the law, this is known as the patient's right to informed consent. Therefore, each patient has the right to be informed of the pros and cons of each test, the course of treatment and the consequences of not proceeding with either the test or treatment. In other words, you have total control over the decision making process.

MAINTAINING YOUR ESTATE

Decisions will have to be made in the event that you are incapacitated as a result of an injury or illness. For example, you will need someone to manage your affairs until you have recovered.

This can be done as follows:

- *Power of Attorney*

  A power of attorney is a legal document that gives an attorney or anyone you choose the authority to act on your behalf. The authority given by the "principal" or the person who signs the power of attorney can be general or specific both in terms of scope and the time frame within which the document is in effect.

  A "specific or general" power of attorney allows you (the principal) to choose someone to manage part or all of your affairs. For example, if you are going on a cruise, you can appoint someone to pay your bills, manage your assets, and in general, keep your affairs in order, until you return. Or if you are selling property, you can give someone the power of attorney to transact the sale on your behalf.

  You have the right to set the limits of the power of attorney, which is outlined in the document. Likewise, you can limit the time in which the person acts on your behalf. The power of attorney automatically ceases upon the death or incapacitation of the principal, and can be revoked by the principal at any time.

Before you sign a power of attorney, you should consult with a lawyer for the following reasons:

o   As with most legal documents, language used in a document is very important. The lawyer should ensure that the document is properly prepared and executed and that you are assigned only those responsibilities that you are comfortable with.

o   The court has no legal control over the power of attorney document. As a result, any damage done to you or your estate, whether intentionally or because of negligence, cannot be prosecuted in the court.

o   The person so assigned as power of attorney is also known as a fiduciary to the principal and is legally obligated to act in the best interest of the principal at all times. In addition, the fiduciary must not mix his assets with that of the principal's. In fact, the he or she is guided by a code of ethics that are enforceable by law.

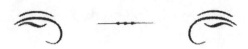

PRE-PLANNING THE LAST GOODBYE

Most of us do not think about death. But someone has to make the necessary arrangements when we die.

The following are some of the things that must be dealt with when that time comes:

- Employing the services of a mortuary

  A mortuary is a place, especially a funeral home, where dead bodies are kept prior to cremation or burial. The services they offer include, collecting the body, embalming (or holding the body in cold storage until the funeral), securing signatures and death certificates, preparation of the body (if there is to be a viewing) and the use of the facility.

  The fee charged by a mortuary varies, and is dependent on the type of services that it offers.

Mortuaries differ in size and "specialty", in the sense that some only cater to certain religious or cultural groups. This diversity means that the family is likely to get the best service available, at the best price if proper planning is done. For example, you can arrange everything yourself, so that all that is required of the family is to put your plan in action.

- *Final Resting Place*

The family also has to choose either cremation or burial. However, this can be specified in your will. If you chose to be buried, it is important that you identify the spot where you would like to be buried. Cemetery plots can be compared to housing lots, the better the view and the "neighbourhood," the higher the cost. You can buy ahead of time, in which case you choose the space you want at the price you can afford.

- *Funeral Arrangements*

By making arrangements ahead of time, you can make you wishes known, thereby relieving your family of an additional burden.

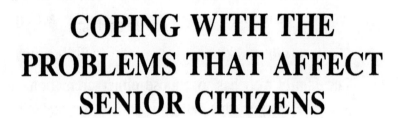

COPING WITH THE PROBLEMS THAT AFFECT SENIOR CITIZENS

Senior citizens face many problems, which tend to become more significant, as they get older. One common problem is abuse.

ABUSE

Senior citizen abuse occurs when an elderly person is not being cared for with the respect and dignity, which is the right of every human being. Neglect can be just as harmful to a senior citizen as physical abuse, and is usually more common. There are many signs that indicate neglect, including weight loss and poor health. In an institution, the presence of bedsores is a good indication that the person is not being moved on a regular basis. Whether, private, institutional, no form of neglect should be ignored.

The rate of abuse of senior citizen is on the increase,

and in most cases is perpetuated by the victim's children, close relatives, in nursing homes or other residential facilities. Most victims are reluctant to discuss the problem out of guilt or fear of retaliation from those who carry out the act. Some physical signs of abuse include unexplained bruises and cuts. Other signs are subtler, ranging from fear of the caregiver to unexplained drowsiness due to excessive sedation. In this instance, it is very difficult to detect that a person is being abused, unless someone actually witnesses the act. In the event that you do, you should notify the police, who will direct you to the proper authorities. It is important to note though, that not all cuts and bruises, fractured or broken limb are signs that the person is being abused, as in some cases the person might have simply fallen from the bed.

You can also discuss the situation with an investigator or social worker. You should be as detailed and specific as possible in your description. Reporting that 'something does not seem right' is not enough justification for an investigation. If the investigator or social worker believes that there is enough (reasonable) evidence that a problem exists, they will conduct an investigation, after which the necessary steps will be taken to remedy the situation. This can range from counselling for the victim and his or her family to finding alternate housing arrangements for the abused person.

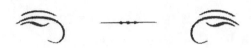

WHEN YOUR SPOUSE IS TERMINALLY ILL

In recent years, a variety of services has been developed to assist in the care of a terminally ill person. Among these are hospice care and grief counselling.

HOSPICE CARE

A hospice is not just a place; it is a philosophy that combines loving care and support with medical assistance, to reduce the pain and suffering of the terminally ill. If a victim decides to explore all possible options in the treatment of the condition, then hospice care is not the best option. However, if the decision is to let the disease run its natural course, then hospice care maybe an appropriate choice, in which case you automatically give up your rights to the use of any life-saving medical technique, or to be resuscitated in the event that you stop breathing. Instead, it is the responsibility of hospice to control pain and provide support.

Hospice care usually begins when a physician has diagnosed a patient as having a terminal illness. It can be at home or in a hospital. In the case of the former, family or friends must be willing and available to undertake the responsibility of being the primary caregiver of the person who is dying. In the case of the latter, many hospices have designated spaces in hospitals in the event that they feel that the victim would be better served in that setting.

The hospice team is made up of the patient's primary care physician, nurses, psychologists and social workers, who assist the patient and family to adjust to or deal with the situation. Sometimes a member of the clergy is made available to those who require such support. Also a minister/pastor or a specially trained volunteer is assigned and his/her job is simply to help all those involved, to deal with the situation.

The services of a hospice do not end when the person dies, as the family members can benefit from grief counselling, which is an important service that is offered by the hospice.

GRIEF COUNSELLING

When a loved one has died, or is dying, it is very important that the survivors get assistance to work through the different emotions that they are experiencing. This usually takes the form of grief, and is expressed by crying, feelings of exhaustion, frustration and emptiness, tightening in the throat, and other physical or emotional sensation. Grief may range from a preoccupation with the memories of happier with the deceased to anger aimed at the deceased for dying.

To this end, psychologists have responded with a service called grief counselling, which may be in the form of a support group made up of the patient's family, group therapy for the widow or widower, or one-on-one sessions with a psychologist or therapist. Whatever its form, the purpose of grief counselling is to help the survivors to deal with their loss or any unresolved issue between them and the deceased, the fear of being alone and to move on with their lives.

Grief counselling programmes may also be offered by hospitals. There are also mental health professionals who are specialists in this area.

If you are interested in additional information, contact your local mental health association, your local chapter of the Cancer Society, church or ask your physician for a referral.

WIDOWHOOD

In addition to grieving, a newly widowed person has many other things to deal with. The following is a short list of tasks that have to be performed by most widows upon the death of their spouse.

- *Funeral arrangements*

  Arrangements must be made, including the funeral service and place of burial, among others.

- *Processing of documents*

  When there is a death, there are many documents that must be processed, including the death certificate (which can be obtained by the mortician). You should ensure that you get several copies of the death certificate, as it will be needed many times in the days and weeks to come. Insurance certificates must be presented to the insurance company so that the claims can be processed. If the surviving spouse is applying for benefits, copies of the marriage certificate will be required. Wills, living trust or other such documents, which come into effect upon the death of the spouse, should be handed over to a lawyer for processing. Deeds and other written evidence of title to property should be at hand in the event that probate becomes necessary.

- *Moving on with your life*

  Obviously, this may be easier said than done. But there comes a time when all the paperwork has been processed, the legal formalities have been completed and grief is beginning to abate. This may be a good time to start a new job or do some volunteer work. You can also join a social club or a center for senior citizens, or in some cases, selling your home and moving closer to your children.

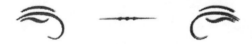

5

MONEY MATTERS
& EMPLOYMENT

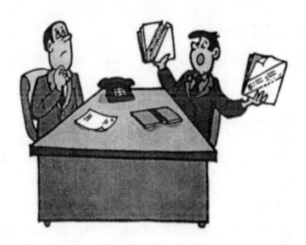

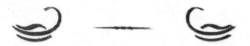

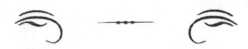

PENSION

A pension is an ancillary benefit of employment (meaning an addition to salary), and is offered by the employer as part of the employment package. There are many different types of pension plans that are offered by the private sector, unions or government agencies.

TYPES OF PENSION PLANS

Pensions generally fall into four categories. They are defined benefit, defined contribution and civil service plan.

- *Defined Benefit*

   These pension plans are probably the most common and are the easiest to understand. Basically you are guaranteed a specific sum of money when you retire. This can either be a certain amount per month for each year of service or the payment can be based on a percentage of your average salary over the years of employment. In other words, the amount given is based on a set formula.

- *Defined contribution*

  Under this type of plan, the exact amount of money that you will receive is not known until you retire. Your employer contributes a specific amount per employee into the pension plan. This money is then invested. When you retire, you are entitled to receive a sum of money, which is determined on the basis of the amount that the employer contributed, in addition to a proportionate share of the interest earned over the years. Sometimes, the employer only guarantees to put in a percentage of profits rather than a specified amount. In this instance, it is called a profit sharing plan. Upon retirement, the employee can choose the method of payment, either monthly or a lump sum.

- *Civil Service Pension Plans*

  If you work in a government agency, you are entitled to receive a pension at the end of your tenure. While each pension scheme may differ, the amount of money you receive is based on the number of years you were employed and an average of your highest income earned over the years. Civil service pension plans also have the following features, which make them particularly attractive, especially when compared to private sector pension plans.

o A cost of living adjustment. Most private pensions do not factor in inflation.

o Full vesting (the right to receive a full pension) after five years rather than ten or more years.

o The right to "roll over " your pension (take it with you) if you move your employment from one government agency to another.

o Early retirement, sometimes as early as the age of 55 years.

o The right to your pension even if you are working elsewhere.

FEATURES TO LOOK FOR IN YOUR PENSION PLAN

Upon retirement, if you are entitled to a pension, you should be aware of the following:

- *Vesting period*

In order to be eligible for pension, you must work for a specific period of time called the vesting period. Once you have worked the specified number of years, you are entitled to receive a full pension upon retirement. If you leave before the time specified, you are partially vested, which means that you will receive only a part of the pension or in some cases, none. Therefore, it is important that you understand the features of your pension plan before you decide to quit or change jobs.

- *Payment of benefits*

  Some plans do not give you an option as to how the benefits are paid out. Others do.

  These choices are as follows:

  o A lump sum payment or monthly payments

  The lump sum payment method is usually very attractive, as you collect a large sum of money at once. In addition, by accepting a lump sum, you are guaranteed to receive all you are entitled upon retirement, but it would be subjected to more tax. If you opt for monthly payments, in the event that you die, all payments could be terminated.

  o Monthly benefits or payments to be passed on to your spouse upon death.

  Most payments cease upon the death of the person · receiving the benefits. However, many plans allow for the transfer of benefits or payments to the spouse (sometimes at

reduced rates) upon the death of the pensioner. A variation of this is to provide a small
benefit or payment to the spouse or other
beneficiary for a specific number of years
after the pensioner's death.

o Early retirement.

Somewhat similar to the early retirement
option offered by social security, in which
the pensioner is given the option to retire
early beneficiaries and receive less benefits
or lower payments.

- *Other benefits.*

Some plans offer health and life insurance coverage,
as well as monthly payments after retirement

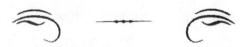

INVESTING

To invest or not to invest is often a dilemma faced each year by many people who retire and suddenly find themselves with a lot of money. Unfortunately, each year many of these persons lose their entire savings in investment plans.

WHAT YOU SHOULD KNOW ABOUT INVESTING

If you intend to invest your money, you should consider the following:

- *Remember who you are*

  Use the knowledge you have learnt over the years. If you have worked extensively in real estate, you might want to invest in that area, rather than in the commodities market. If you are unsure about what you are doing, do not do it!

- *Have enough cash available to handle an emergency*

It does not mean that you should keep large sums of money at home or on your person. It may mean, however, that you invest it in a 30 to 90 day in a savings institution for a specified period of time in what is called a certificate of deposit (CD). Certificate of deposits earn a slightly higher rate of interest than a regular passbook savings account. However, they attract a penalty if the money is withdrawn before the period expires. By rolling over your CD (reinvesting into another CD upon maturity) you will increase your principal and maintain liquidity

- *Remember "the sleep factor."*

  That is, will you lose sleep because of the investment? If you are investing money you really cannot afford to lose or the risk is too high, you are better off playing it safe.

- *Decide what you want from your investment.*

  Some investments are designed to increase in value over the years, while others are designed to produce a steady flow of income. Some, of course, do both. Before you invest, decide what you want and ensure that the investment selected is suited to your needs.

- *Decide whether or not you are going to use a financial adviser.*

  A financial adviser's job is to analyze your financial

needs, such as income requirements, tax liabilities and gives you advice on the best way to manage or invest your money.

It is important to note that some financial advisers are paid a commission from the proceeds of your investments. Others may charge you a straight or hourly fee, after which you may still have to pay a commission on every investment. Ensure that you agree on a method of payment before you his or her services.

INVESTMENT OPPORTUNITIES

- *Certificates of Deposits or Money Market Accounts* are services offered by banks and savings and loans institution at higher interest rates than passbook accounts.

  Risk: Low

  Earning potential: Varies, depending on the economy.

- *Government Bonds* are promissory notes from government agencies that become due on a specific date and earn a specific rate of interest. They are bought and sold on the bond market.

Risk: The value of the bonds fluctuates and is subject to inflation. However, if you keep them long enough, the face value will be paid when they become due. Treasury bonds are secure. Some municipal bonds may be less so.

Earning potential: If the value rises after you purchase the bonds and then you sell, you make money. However, the most positive feature of government bonds, especially treasury bonds, is that they are income secure, that is, the amount of interest you earn per month will not vary, despite the market value. Municipal bonds are tax free, but usually pay a lower interest rate.

- *Corporate Bonds*, like government bonds, are promissory notes. However, the money is borrowed from the private sector rather than from the public sector. As with government bonds, the face value of the bond is established along with the interest rate.

  Risk: Dependent on the corporation issuing the bonds.

  Earning potential: Usually the greater the risk, the greater the income and vice versa. The monthly payment terms will vary, so be sure to read the fine print.

- *Stocks* are ownership interests in corporations. They are generally bought and sold in the various stock markets and often pay income based on profits to shareholders called dividends.

  Risk: High. The stock market is very volatile and even an experienced player, not to mention a novice, can get frustrated. If you buy on margin (where you put up part of the money and the brokerage house loans you the rest), the risk is even greater since the stock may be sold if the market goes down in order to protect the loan.

  Earning potential: Can be high if you buy low and sell high or vice versa. Also, if you get stocks in a good, solid company, you can make good returns on your investment.

- *Mutual Funds* take smaller investments and pool them together into a very large fund, which is then used to invest in specific areas of the financial market. The advantage of mutual funds is professional management and its ability to diversify holdings so that losses are minimized.

  Risk: The risk is high or low depending on the nature of the investments and the quality of the management.

  Earning potential: You can earn a good return on

mutual fund investments if it is properly managed.

- *Trust Deeds* are loans to owners of real estate and is "secured" by the real estate itself.

  Risk: Trust Deeds (TDs) can be safe if the real estate has been accurately appraised, contains sufficient equity to cover the loan in the event of sale and is fully insured for fire or other loss. However, they can be a risk especially if you have a second or third TD, which means that you collect behind the first creditors in the event of default. If you are not familiar with real estate transactions, it is best that you do not invest in TDs.

  Earning potential: Trust Deeds can earn a good return depending on the interest rate charged.

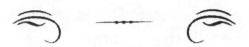

EMPLOYMENT

A difficulty that many senior citizens face, is finding interesting and gainful employment after retirement. The reality is that many employers simply do not employ senior citizens. So many of the jobs offered to them are either menial in nature, sporadic or so low-paying that they may not be worth the effort.

However, there are jobs that are available that will make use of your specific skill and years of experience.

TIPS ON HOW TO FIND A GOOD JOB

In order to get the job that is best suited to your needs, consider the following:

- *Take an inventory of yourself*

  Honestly assess your physical, mental and emotional conditions and what you are looking for in a job. Get a good idea of what it is you can and cannot do and what you want and do not want to do. Ask yourself the following questions to prepare yourself for your search:

o **"How much money do I need to earn?"** Your financial situation will probably determine the type of job you choose.

o **"What type job would I like?"** And "What job will I be willing to accept?" The answers to these two questions will define the parameters of your search.

o **"How far from home am I willing to work?"** The answer to this question will depend on such matters as your health and physical abilities, your responsibilities at home and the availability of transportation.

o **"What days and how many hours am I willing to work?"** A job that requires you to work weekends when you are not willing to do so clearly is not worth applying for. If you are willing to work unusual hours, your search may prove to be easier.

o **"What is my experience?"** The answer to this question involves far more than job title or description; it's the essence of what you actually have done and can still do. You must be prepared to tell the prospective employer everything about yourself and your capabilities.

o **"What are my skills?"** If you are strong in organizational skills, be prepared to tell the interviewer and have examples to back up your claim.

o **"Why do I want to work?"** Many employers may not understand why you want to work. There is nothing wrong with saying you need the money. You can also say you enjoy the feeling of being productive and contributing to a worthwhile cause.

● *Realize that you might need help*

Many seniors are unprepared for the difficulties associated with job hunting. Although they may have worked for a long time, does not mean that they are experienced in seeking a new job. Do not hesitate to join a support group. After all, the enthusiasm of others can go a long way in motivating you and giving you the confidence you may need.

● *Be prepared to take no for an answer*

That does not mean that you are passive. You simply have to accept the "no" until you get a "yes." If you are serious in your desire, you will not give up until you achieve your goal.

- *Learn to read the signs*

    There is a difference between being aggressive and wasting your time. Here are some signs, which will help you decide when to go for it or to move on:

'Buy' Signs	'Bye' Signs
"What experience do you have?" This question indicates interest and an open mind.	"Send a resume." This means, I do not have the guts to Say I'm not interested. (Send your resume anyway , they might mean it.)
"Where have you worked before?"	"Come in and apply." See above.
"Tell me about your last job."	"You're not qualified." It's going to be difficult to change this person's mind.
What can you do for me?'	"We already have someone else in mind." In other words, we do not want to hire you .

- Do not take rejection personally

  Remember, being denied is part of the process. Do not take it personally if a prospective employer turns down your request for employment. If you allow a "no" to lower your self-esteem, you might communicate this negativity in your next interview session.

- *Search for the jobs*

  Contrary to popular belief, the classified section in the newspaper is not necessarily the best place to look for a job. In fact, the classifieds are often the last place employers advertise to fill a vacant position. Do not be afraid to telephone companies or walk in and apply for a job. Set yourself a goal of at least two interviews per week, go out and make it happen. Send thank you notes to the interviewer even if you were rejected and do follow up checks at places where you sensed interest.

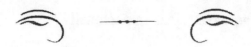

INSURANCE POLICIES

TIPS ON BUYING HEALTH INSURANCE POLICIES

The following are some important factors that you should take into consideration when you are buying an insurance policy.

- *Pre-existing illness exclusions*

  Many policies exclude from coverage, prior illnesses or conditions for which you have been recently treated, either for the duration of the policy or for a specific period of time after the policy goes into effect. For example, if you had cancer, did radiation therapy three months prior to your purchase of the policy and further treatment is required, if a pre-existing illness exclusion clause is in the document, then your policy would not cover this treatment.

- *Indemnity payments*

  An indemnity benefit pays a specific amount of

money for each day you are hospitalized. The amount is fixed and will not increase even if your medical costs increase. As a result, it can be affected by inflation.

- *Elimination periods*

  Rather than pay your medical cost from the day you enter the hospital, you are subjected to an "elimination period" which can be up to a period of one week. If the elimination period is longer, you may never see the monies you were promised when you took out the insurance policy.

- *Renewability clauses*

  Do not sign a policy that is "optionally renewable." It means that the company can decline to renew it at the end of the policy year if it so desires. You should choose a policy that allows you to renew it as long or as often as you want to.

SENIOR CITIZENS AND LIFE INSURANCE

Most senior citizens are familiar with the type of life insurance policy where the insurance company hopes that you live, and you hope that you die. If you live, they collect premiums and pay you nothing (except under "whole life" policies where you build up an equity in your policy). If you die, the life insurance company pays your beneficiaries the face value of the life insurance policy.

Life insurance has traditionally been purchased to protect the family in the event that the breadwinner(s) dies. However, by the time they reach retirement age, many senior citizens either have no policies, or they have long since cashed them in.

Most life insurance companies do not want to offer life insurance to people 70 years and older because the mortality rate is relatively higher at that age. For example, the death rate for a 70 year old could be a thousand times higher than that of a 30 year old. However, there are some companies that market specifically to seniors. If the deal is too good to be true, check the benefits. They are usually limited.

Here is a comparison of the claim and actual benefit or term of a typical company taken directly from their sales brochure:

CLAIM 1: Affordable term life insurance as little as a monthly premium of J$181.70 (US$3.95) per J$46,000 (US$1000) of insurance.

TERMS: if you are a man, the J$181.70 would only

168

pay J$27,600 (US$600) upon your death by natural causes if you die at age 64 years, and only J$18,400 (US$400) if you die between the ages of 70 and 74. If you die because of an accident at age 70, the benefit would only be J$150,880 (US$3,280), which is hardly enough to pay for a decent burial. For a 70 year old man to receive a natural death benefit of J$64,400 (US$1400), he would have to pay a premium of J$908.50 (US$19.75) per month. Benefits are slightly higher for women. If a husband and wife, both between the ages 70-74 want to be covered for J$64,400 (US$1,400) and J$92,000(US$2000) respectively, the premium would be almost J$1840 (US$40) per month or J$22,080 (US$480) per year.

CLAIM 2: No medical exam required; no questions asked!

TERMS: They can offer this "benefit" because if you die of natural causes in the first two years, the only benefit you will receive is the sum total of the premium that you have already paid.

CLAIM 3: Up to J$2,024,000 (US$44,000) in total benefits, depending on age and sex.

TERMS: There is a distinction between natural death and accidental death. In order to receive "total benefits," the death must be ruled an accident. The only person who could qualify for the above amount, is a woman between the ages of 40-44 who spent J$917.70(US$19.95) per month on the policy and who dies an accidental death. A natural death would pay only J$441,600 (US$9,600). A woman who pays the same premium who dies accidentally at age 68 would receive J$966,000 (US$21,000). However, if she dies of natural causes, she would receive only J$138,000 (US$3,000). There is another catch. An exclusion under the accidental death benefit is made for accidents resulting "directly or indirectly from: any disease or bodily infirmity...." In other words, if you fall down a flight of stairs because you are old or sick, your beneficiaries might not be able to collect the larger accidental death benefit.

Please note this is not to influence anyone to choose either of these policies. It should be used as a guideline when you are considering life insurance coverage.

LaVergne, TN USA
31 July 2010
191538LV00002B/7/P